MEDICATED DIET OF TRADITIONAL CHINESE MEDICINE

中华药膳

Chief Editor Hou Jinglun
Associate Editor-in-chief Zhao Xin Li Weidong
Editor Liu Jianxin Geng Chun-e
Li Guohua Li Shaohua

主 编 侯景伦
副主编 赵 昕 李卫东
编 委 刘建新 耿春娥 李国华 李少华

BEIJING SCIENCE & TECHNOLOGY PRESS
北京科学技术出版社

First Edition 1994
ISBN 7-5304-1735-5/R・309

MEDICATED DIET OF TRADITIONAL CHINESE MEDICINE
Chief Editor: Hou Jinglun
Associate Editor-in-Chief: Zhao Xin Li weidong
Editor: Liu Jianxin Geng Chun-e Li Guohua Li Shaohua
Published by: Beijing Science & Technology Press

Distributed by
China International Book Trading Corporation
35 Chegongzhuang Xilu, Beijing, 100044, China
P. O. Box 399 Beijing, China

Printed in the People's Republic of China

PREFACE

Medicated diet of Traditional Chinese medicine (TCM) has a long history. It is an important composite part of the theoretical system of the TCM. Under the guidance of basic theory of TCM, the dietetic Chinese drugs are compatible to base on differentiation of symptoms and signs. It' s a synthetic subject, for preventing and curing diseases, building up one' s health and prolonging one' s life etc.

The medicated diet of TCM is paid attention in the developing history of the TCM science. The famous pharmacologist of past ages studied the basic theory and principal of this subject from different respect s and refert to lay stress on the whole and select medicated diet on the basis of differential diagnosis; suitable for both prevention and treatment; outstanding efficiency; and good in taste and conventent for taking etc. On the centenary, as characteristic of the theoretical system, as a result of the continual development of the productive force and sicientific technology, the idea of the human traditional treatment and health care tend to the method of the natural treatment as well. Personnel of the different department has paid close attention to the dietetic treatment of TCM on its taste, colour, odour and the dual nature of medicine and food.

Especially in the wake of the China reform and opening to the outside world, TCM frequently exchanges to the out—side world, the Chinese dietetic treatment has begun to go to the world too. Various medicated diet foods and health care drinks have been sold at the international market, medicated diet dinning—halls have been seted up in some countries. In addition, a great number of friends are greatly interested in it, hoping to develop acondemic exchanges and technical and economic cooperation in this repect, so as to promot the internationaization of the dietotheraphy of TCM.

TCM, which dates back to ancient times, has a unique and Profound theoretical system. The greater Part of its terminology has particular denotations, and is matter—of—factly difficult to understand and translate. Inaccuracies in the library, therefore, are unavoidable. I hope that my friends in the TCM circle will oblige me with timely corrections.

Chief Editor
Hou Jinglun
Mid-autumn Fastival, 1994

CONTENTS

Chapter one

General Introduction

The dietetic therapeutics of Traditional Chinese Medicine (TCM) is a synthetic subject which prepare the dietetic Chinese drugs to base on differentiation of symptoms and signs under the basic theoretical guidance of TCM. It is an important composite part of the theoretical system of TCM. Not only has it the efficiency of medicine but also the delicacy of food, and can be used to prevent and cure diseases, build up one's health and prolong one's life.

Section 1

Origin and Development

The science of dietetic treatment in TCM, which emerged with man's practice in medical hygiene, has a long history. Expositions concerning dietetic Chinese drugs and dietetic treatment can be found in almost any literature in TCM through the ages. The ancient legend "Shennong Tastes a Hundred Grasses" shows that early in remote antiquity the Chinese nation had begun to explore the function of food and medicaments, hence the saying "TCM and medicated diet both originate from the practice and experience in daily life."

In the Shang Dynasty, one thousand six hundred years B.C., the emperor Shang Tang had special disscussions with his prime minister Yi Yin on Chinese cuisine, involving a great deal about the cooking of food and drink. In the Zhou Dynasty, it is recorded in Zhou Ceremony that royal doctors were divided into four kinds. One of them was dietetic doctors who were in charge of emperor's health care and health preservation, preparing diets for him.

In the Yellow Emperor's Internal Classic, a medical classic in TCM, which appeared approximately in the Warring States Period, we can find theoretical exposition of dietotherapy in it, which emphasized "compatibility of viscera with the property and taste of food," and listed some foods and several medicated diet prescriptions that could tonify and nourish the viscera and be compatible with the viscera. In Shennong's Herbal Classic, which was published approximately in about the Qin and Han periods and is the extant earliest monography on materia medica, many sorts of medicaments which are dietetic Chinese drugs was recorded. Zhang Zhongjing, a famous physician in the East Han Dynasty, who wrote the book Treatise on Febrile and Miscellaneous Diseases, realized the action of dietotherapy during the rehabilitation from diseases and put forward the concept of "dietetic incompatibility," such as "The pungent should be abstained from liver diseases, the salt from heart diseases, the sour from spleen diseases, bitter from lung diseases," etc., and some noted medicated diet recipes were recorded, such as Soup of Chinese Angelica Root, Fresh Ginger and Mutton, Soup of Lily Bulb and Yolk, etc., all of which now still have important values.

Sun Simiao, a famous physician in the Tang Dynasty who wrote the two books Prescriptions Worth a Thousand Gold for Emergencies and A Supplement to Essential Prescriptions Worth a Thousand Gold for Emergencies discussed such questions as dietetic treatment, dietetic treatment for senile health care and health preservation etc., in his book, and those two books recorded a substantial prescriptons of medicated diet.

The book Dietotherapy of Materia Medica by Meng Xian in the Tang Dynasty is the exant earliest monograph on dietetic treatment, it has a great influence on later generations.

According to history books, up to the period of the Sui and Tang Dynasties about more than sixty kinds of books on dietetic treatment had been published. But unfortunately most of them are lost. Thereafter, works was daily increasing, which researched and discussed in the dietetic treatment respect, such as the book Principles of Correct Diet, a monograph on medicated diet, by Hu Sihui, a royal doctor in the Yuan Dynasty; the book Recipe of sui Xiju written by Wang Shixiong, A famous physician in the Qing Dynasty, introduced over 300 species belonging to 7 phyla of medicated food and drink in his book.

The book Analysis of Food and Drink for Treatment of Disease by Zhang Mu, and the book Cook Book of Suiyuan by Yuan mei, etc., these monographys on medicated diet treatment in the Qin Dynasty varied in characteristics.

Now because of the development of economy and the continuous rising of the people's living standard, the research and exploitation of medicated diet is more and more valued by the personnel of different departments, and a number of works about medicated diet with distinctive traditional features have been colleted and published one after another. For example, the books Principles of Correct Diet by Hu Sihui in the Yuan Dynasty and Recipe of Sui Xiju by Wang shixiong in Qing Dynasty, etc. The publishing of these books will play an important role in carrying on the experiences in ancient medicated diet.

In short, a comprehensive survey of the ancient and modern times shows that the dietetic therapeutics of TCM has had a long and venerable history and is well established with new ideas and developments at each generation. With its substantial content, it will certainly make greater contributions to the health of mankind.

Section 2

Characteristics

The characteristics of the medicated diet in TCM are as follows:

1)Making Up Diet on the Basis of Differentiation of Syndromes.

The dietetic treatment should be guided by the basic theories of TCM, based on the differentiation of syndromes and the correct diagnosis. When prescribing medicated diet, we should first make an overall analysis of the patient's physical and health condition, the nature of his illness, the season he got ill in and the geographical condition, etc., form a judgement on the type of syndrome; then decide on corresponding principles for dietetic therapy and select suitable medicated diet. Dietetic treatment of each case, the dietetic recipe or formula should strictly follow the principles, and the principles should be confirmed under the guidance of theories. Generally, satisfactory result can be achieved through the above mentioned procedure.

But dietotherapy should be rational in prescription to avoid the negative aspect and obtain the positive aspect. In True Understanding of Materia Medica, the author pointed out: "Taking foods and treating diseases with medicines share the same principle: the compatibility benefits man's viscera and thus prevents him from or cures him of diseases and protects his life, while incompatibility damages his viscera and thus worsens his disease or even hastens his death."

That is why emphasis should be placed on differentiation of syndromes in therapy with diet. If it is abused, tonification and purgation may be mistaken for excess syndrome and deficiency syndrome, which, surely, will lead to adverse result.

2)Balancing the Five Flavours and Four Natures: Dietetic Chinese drugs refer to Chinese medicinal edibles having the functions of nourishing the human body and keeping fit as well as preventing and curing diseases. They belong to the category of traditional Chinese drugs, so the theory of the nature of traditional Chinese drugs is also applicable to dietetic Chinese drugs.

Like common traditional Chinese drugs, dietetic Chinese drugs are different from one another in nature and taste. According to TCM theories, the five tastes, namely sour, bitter, sweet, acrid and salty, and the four nature, namely cold, hot, warm and cool.

Different nature and flavour of dietetic Chinese drugs have different curative effect. What's more, the natures and flavours of dietetic Chinese drugs are interrelated with the five viscera, selection and mixing of certain dietetic Chinese drugs possessing different natures or tastes may exert different effect on the five viscera.

Zhang Zhongjing, a physician in the middle of 2nd-3rd century, said: "Dietetic tastes may exert active effect on health recovery, or exert negative effect on health. Proper application of them will be beneficial; improper application, harmful." It can be said that selecting dietetic Chinese drugs according to the properties of dietetic Chinese drugs and characteristics of viscera is also an important principle in treatment with medicated diet.

First of all, TCM holds that dietetic Chinese drugs are different in tastes. The five tastes each have an affinity for a specific zang-organ. This is what is meant by "as each individual has a preference for a specific kind of colour, smell or taste, each flavour goes to a specific zang-organ." ("Discussion on Viscera-State Doctrine". Chapter 9 of Plain Questions) Of the five tastes "sour is attributed to the liver, bitter to the heart, sweet to the spleen, pungent to the lung, and salty to the kidney. "("Discussion on Five Flavours", Chapter 63 of Miraculous Pivot) So only diet with a proper pattern of the five tastes can keep "the bone tough, muscles soft and pliable, qi and blood smooth in circulation and body surface dense and maintain the functions of the five zang-organs coordinate and harmonious. Conversely, persistent addiction to a certain tastes will lead to its accumulation within the body, "which, in the course of time, will result in pathogenic excess of qi in a certain zang-organ, "ultimately giving rise to dysfunction of viscera. Chapter 3 of Plain Questions stated: "The five zang-organs depend upon the five flavours for their function; excess of the five tastes brings damage to the five zang-organs. Oversour causes the liver-qi to be in excess, which overacts on the spleen and results in the exhaustion of the spleen-qi. Oversalty brings damage to the bone and causes the muscles to wither and the heart-qi to be in depression. Oversweet causes the heart-qi to be in distention and fullness, the face to be black in colour, and the kidney-qi to be in disequilibrium. Overbitter causes the spleen-qi to be in dryness, giving rise to distention and fullness of the stomach. Overpungent causes the muscles to be in relaxation and debility and the spirit to be impaired. "

On the basis of analysis of dietetic Chinese drugs conducted over a long period of life and medical practice, our forefathers advised people "to eat the five cereals to nourish the vital-qi of the five zang-organs, with the five fruits, the five meats, and the five vegetables as supplements. "("Discussion on Relation between Viscera-qi and Seasons", Chapter 22 of Plain Questions)

The five cereals: rice, sweet; sesame, sour; soy beans, salty; wheat, bitter; broomcorn millet, acrid.

The five fruits: date, sweet; plum, sour; chestnut, salty; apricot, bitter; peach, acrid.

The meat of the five animals: beef, sweet; dog meat, sour; pork, salty; mutton, bitter; chicken, acrid.

The five vegetables: cluster mallow, sweet; chives, sour; leaves of pulse plant, salty; macrostem onion, bitter; scallion, acrid.

(All the above are seen in Discussion on the "Five Flavours", Chapter 63 of Miraculous pivot)

In addition, The dietetic Chinese drugs are different in nature: cold, hot, warm or cool. Goose eggs, for example, are warm, chicken eggs are neutral and duck eggs cool; beef and mutton are warm and pork is neutral. The four natures of dietetic Chinese drugs have the functions of recovering the imbalance between yin and yang within the body. Here is a brief list of common dietetic Chinese drugs that belong to hot-warm type, cold-cool type and neutral type respectively.

Hot-warm type: mutton, beef, dog meat, chicken, pigeon, sheep milk, cow milk, goose eggs, carp, yellow croaker, hairfail, tortoise, crucian carp, snakeheaded fish, cuttlefish, brown sugar and refined sugar, peanut, sesame, soybean, rice, wheat flour, date, longan, litchi, mandarin orange, tangerine, orange, apple, green onion, garlic, Chinese chives, coriander, day lily, sweet potato, ginger, chilli, Chinese prickly ash, pepper and so on.

Neutral type: pork, pork liver, chicken egg, jelly-fish skin, tremella, water chestnut, red bean, pea, radish, lotus seed, lotus root, Chinese yam, seed of Job's tears, spinage, carrot, tomato, Chinese cabbage, fresh kidney bean and so on.

Cold-cool type: duck, duck eggs, honey, seaweed, kelp, mung bean, white gourd, water melon, towel gourd, cucumber, lettuce, bamboo shoots, black fungus, banana, persimmon, pear, bean curd and so on.

Besides, diet should have a proper pattern in temperature; it should neither be too hot nor too cold. Main Notes on Protecting Life says: "Whatever diet that is too hot in temperature injures the bone and whatever diet that is too cold in temperature injures the tendon. Diet must not be taken as hot as burns the lips or as cold as freezes the teeth."

3) Preparing Medicated Diet in Accordance with the Physique of an Individual:

The dietetic Chinese drugs are different in tastes, natures, channel tropisms, and in efficiencies and indications. Therfore, these medicated diets which prepare with dietetic Chinese drugs are usually used to accord the difference of human being in conditions of health:

Those who are of wood-fire constitution should eat these medicated diets which prepare with the light dietetic Chinese drugs with moistening effect, such as fruits, vegetables, millet, beans, milk, eggs, and cautiously have food that produces heat and promotes fire, such as Chinese prickly ash, chilli, beef, mutton, dog meat. Those who are of the phlegm-dampness constitution should eat those medicated diets which prepare with the light dietetic Chinese drugs that removes dampness by diuresis, such as fruits, vegetables, millets, and sparingly have the greasy diet that produces phlegm and promotes dampness, such as fat, milk products. Those who are of yang-deficiency constitution should eat these medicated diets which prepare with these dietetic Chinese drugs that have an acrid nature and a warm property, such as fish, meat of birds and domestic fowls, beef, mutton as well as ginger, chilli, and it is not appropriate for them to take cold meat dishes, cold drinks or fruits.

Besides, as "the yin-qi of people decreases by half at the age of forty, the aged are frequently in such conditions as excess of yang-qi and insufficiency of yin-essence." Therefore, it is appropriate for the aged to have the neutral and tonic, light and invigorating yin medicated diets.

4) Protecting the Spleen and Stomach: One of the characteristics is that take physiology and pathology of the spleen and stomach into consideration in medicated diet therapy, through which the spleen and stomach are then nursed, health recovered. As the spleen and stomach provide the material basis of the acquired constitution function as the important organs in digesting food and absorbing and transporting food essence and serve as the source of qi and blood formation. When the spleen-qi and stomach-qi are vigorous, qi and blood are abundantly transformed, and the five zang-organs are then nourished, patients are easier to recover, otherwise deficiency and impairment of the spleen-qi and stomach, poor appetite are sure to hinder treatment with medicated diet.

Section 3

Points for Attention of Dietetic Treatment

1) Proper Cooking

Dietetic Chinese drugs should be chosen carefully and seriously. First of all, cleanness-selecting should be carried out so as to ensure that the drugs and food to be used are clean, pure and dustless, and none of them is mildewed or rotten. The next thing deserving attention is the purity of color and flavor, the beautiful appearance and good quality of the materials and food. Take Chinese-date as an example. Those which are big, purplish red, with plenty of flesh, smooth and not moth-eaten should be used; otherwise, they are of poor quality and should not be used. Take wolfberry fruit (Fructus Lycii) as another example. Those with big grains, plenty of flesh, few seeds, red in color and soft should be used; otherwise, they are of poor quality and should not be used.

In order to ensure the desired result of dietetic Chinese drugs it is necessary, too, for the drugs and food to be processed. Some have to be cut into pieces, cubes, sections, or to be shreded; some have to be ground into powder; and some have to be processed according to the processing requirements for Chinese drugs. For example, parched hawthorn fruit (Fructus Crataegi) can strengthen the spleen and promote digestion; while parched hawthorn fruit charcoal can not only strengthen the spleen and promote digestion, but also stop diarrhea. Some drugs, such as prepared aconite root (Radix Aconiti Praeprata), Jiang ban xia (a kind of prepared pinellia during the preparation of which a decoction of ginger is used), must be processed before they are used so as to reduce their toxicity or side effects.

Cooking techniques must be taken into consideration to prepare good medicated diet. Besides the colour, the fragrance, the taste and the shape that the food cooked in common ways have attention must be paid, when dietetic Chinese drugs is being cooked , to retain as much as possible its nutrition and effective constituents in order to bring into full play its functions of treatment and health care. The main purpose of cooking dietetic Chinese drugs with proper condiments is to maintain the special properties of the original juice and flavor of food and Chinese drugs so that their nature and flavor might be combined closely. As a result, not only does the medicated diet have good colour, fragrance, taste and shape, thus arousing the appetite, but also the treatment of disease and health care are brought into play. Common edible Chinese drugs and those with no improper flavor(or their fine powder)can be cooked together with food; if the drugs to be used are too many or have distinctly improper flavor, they can be wrapped in gauze and cooked along with food, and by doing so, the property of the drugs can go into the food or the soup; the drugs must be sifted out before it is taken. Medicated diet can also be prepared first by decocting Chinese drugs, sifting the liquid from the drugs; then by pouring the liquid into the food being cooked, and cooking them until the medicated diet is done.

As the Chinese people differ in habits of diet, the methods of cooking medicated diet vary. For example, in the light of its form and process, medicated diet can be divided into the fresh juice, medicated tea, drink, medicated wine, decoction, medicated gruel, honey extract, medicated pancake, cooked dishes, etc. But the genaral principle is that every effort should be made to minimize the loss and destruction of nutrients and cook medicated diet such that it is easy to digest and absorb.

In addition, the preparing medicated diet should vary in accordance with the conditions of an individual. For the aged, who are weak in masticatory and digestive functions, food should be cooked fine and soft. This is just what is meant by Chen Zhi of the Song Dynasty said in his work A New Book for prolonging Life of Parents: "Generally, the aged should take diet that is warm or hot, cooked and soft and refrain from glutinous, tough, raw or cold food."

2)Compatibility and Incompatibility of Dietetic Treatment .

As for invigoration and benefit in the four seasons, medicated diet should be prepared regularly in conformity with the changs of the four seasons.

During the three months of spring, it is getting warmer, everything on earth comes to life and the human liver-qi is in the right time to grow and develop. Therefore, "in spring man should eat more sweet food than sour food to nourish the spleen-qi," (Treatise on Health Preservation and Cultivation, by Qiu Chuji, the Yuan Dynasty).

During the three months of summer, it is burning hot and the human digestive function decreases; man should take this medical diet that is light and easy to digest, "shunning greasy and tough food." (A Book Compiled for the Taiping Emperor, Volume DCCXX, by Li Fang et al., the Song Dynasty). Special care must be taken to eat frequently nutritious fruits and vegetables.

During the three months of autumn, the yang-qi weakens while the yin-qi grows; it is getting cool; and so people must not be gluttonous cold and cool medicated diet, to prevent impairment of the spleen and stomach. Water melon, for example, can "clear away summer-heat and relieve excessive thirst," (Everyday Materia Medica, by Wu Rui, the Yuan Dynasty) hence the name "Natural White Tiger Decoction (Tiansheng Baihu Tang)—a heat-clearing agent." But after the beginning of autumn, it must not be eaten frequently, lest it should damage the yang-qi of the spleen and stomach. Li Shizhen of the Ming Dynasty said in Compendium of Materia Medica: "Water melon and muskmelon are cold in nature. Ordinary people think them relieving and refreshing and seek momentary satisfaction from them, without knowing that they impair the spleen and promote dampness."

During the three months of winter, which is the coldest season of all, yin-qi is in excess while yang-qi is insufficient. According to TCM theories, in winter everything on earth hides and yang-qi of the human body lies low accordingly. After the Winter Solstice, however, yang-qi begins to rise again and, in hiding, exist active signs of life; thus it is the best time for the persons who are constantly weak to tone up the body. The key lies in taking dietetic tonics, i. e., to make up for the weakness and rectify the relative deviation of yin or yang with the tonifying effect of specific foods. There are so many good dietetic tonics that one can choose the best and take. "Beef has a sweet flavour and can be used to reinforce the spleen. The spleen and stomach provide the material basis for the acquired qi and blood; to tonify the spleen and stomach means to tonify all." (Fundamentals in Compiling Medical Works, by Wang Fu, the Qing Dynasty) Mutton, sweet in flavour and hot in nature, can be used to invigorate and restore qi and warm the middle-jiao and the lower-jiao. Chicken, sweet in flavour and slightly warm in nature, can warm the middle-jiao, invigorate qi, replenish the vital essence and marrow; they are suited to all those who suffer from consumption and emaciation. Plain duck, sweet in flavour and slightly cool in nature, can nourish the yin of the five zang-organs and remove fever due to consumptive diseases; it is suited to all those who have always suffered from severe deficiency of yin. "

Therefore, it is better to take medicated diet with dispelling effect in spring, medicated diet capable of clearing away heat in summer, medicated diet that is moderate in nature in autumn and medicated diet with nourishing and invigorating effect in winter.

On the other hand, as for diseases in the five viscera, it is to advisable avoid things acrid in flavor for liver diseases, things bitter in flavor for lung disease, things salty in flavor for both heart and kidney diseases and things sweet and sour in flavor for spleen and stomach diseases. As for the patient's physical condition, those who are weak should take invigorating medicated diet, avoid that with dispersing or purging effect; those who are strong should not take more than needed invigorating medicated diet that is warm in nature; those who are yang deficient should take medicated diet with warming and invigorating effect, avoid food that is salty in flavor and cold in nature; while those who are yin deficient should take medicated diet that nourishes yin, avoid food that is acrid in flavor and hot in nature. As for the nature of disease, medicated diet that is cold and cool in nature should be used for heat syndromes, and medicated diet that is acrid in flavor or hot in nature should be avoided; medicated diet that is warm or hot in nature should be used for cold syndromes, and food that is salty in flavor and cold in nature should be avoided. Those who are troubled with weakness of the spleen and stomach, or indigestion should avoid greasy food and drink.

In addition, there are also some incompatibilities of drugs in prescriptions recorded in ancient literature. For example, coptis root (Rhizoma Coptidis), platycodon root (Radix platycodi), smoked plum (Fructus Mume) are incompatible with pork; turtle, with three-coloured amaranth (Amaranthus); ginseng (Radix Ginseng), with radish (Radix Raphani) and so on. Now although there is no experimental evidence, attention should be paid when medicated diet is used.

3) Right Application of Medicated Diet

The medicated diet in traditional Chinese dietotherapy stresses that people should take it regularly. Generally, it should be taken one time, twice in accordance with the function of digestive organs. Because the mixed food generally stays in the stomach for 4-5 hours and it takes some times for the digestive organs to recover their functions.

Meanwhile, for the different physiological and pathological conditions, the needs of medicated diet should be varied. Under the physiological conditions, because in the day man has to work, and thus consumes more energy, and metabolism is more vigorous, more medicated diet is to be taken, while less in the night, especially at sleep. The amount of activities is reduced to minimum, the metabolism is slow. Under special conditions, it should be varied in accordance with the physique of an individual.

Take the aged and children for example. As they are weak in the spleen and stomach, they should have many meals but little food at each so as to benefit digestion and absorption. Under the pathological conditions, such as abnormal emotional changes affect the digesting and absorbing functions of the stomach and spleen. Thus it is inadvisable for man to take food in wild joy, violent rage, great terror and abrupt fright. Li Yu of the Qing Dynasty said: "In anger, it is easy to swallow food but hard to digest it while in sorrow it is hard to swallow and digest; therefore, it is advisable to wait until it subsides. Food, whenever it is taken, should be taken at a time so that it can be easily digested. Eating food late and digesting it would be better than eating it early but being unable to digest it. Indigestion means trouble while good digestion makes man free from worry." Accordingly, he advised "not to take food in weariness" and suggested that "it is inadvisable to take food whenever a mode of emotion begins to develop." (Volume VI, The Collected Works of Li Weng)

In addition, take the differentiation of disease nature for example, patients suffering from chronic deficiency symptoms should accord their physical condition to take medicated diet regularly at small dosages and with perseverance; that is, in a way it is taken little by little without a let-up, and a lot of benefit is assured to result after a long period of time.

In the final analysis, the medicated diet therapy should be in right amount and moderation.

Chapter Two

Dietetic Chinese Drugs

Dietetic Chinese drugs also known as"edible Chinese drugs","dietetic materia medica"or "medicinal food" refer to Chinese medicinal edibles having the functions of nourishing the human body and keeping fit as well as preventing and curing diseases. They are characterized by the dual nature of medicine and food.

In accordance with the main efficiencies of dietetic Chinese drugs, they are divided into seventeen groups, such as drugs for treating exterior syndromes, heat—clearing drugs, purgative drugs and tonics etc. , but only 130 kinds will be discussed in this chapter.

Section 1

Drugs for Treating Exterior Syndromes

The kind of drugs whose principal effect is to disperse pathogenic factors from the superficiality of the body and relieve exterior syndromes belongs to the category of dietetic Chinese drugs for treating exterior syndromes.

Most drugs in this class are acrid in flavour. They can expel pathogenic factors from the superficiality of the body or relieve exterior syndromes by diaphoresis. Their indications are exterior syndromes due to affection by exopathogens. Some of the drugs also have the effects of promoting the dispersing function of the lung, relieving cough and asthma, relieving pain, promoting skin eruption, and inducing diuresis to reduce edema, and can be used to treat cough or dyspnea due to impaired dispersion of the lung — qi, arthralgia due to wind — dampness, measles, German measles, edema and so on.

They should be chosen in accordance with different syndromes. Other classes of drugs such as those for resolving sputum to arrest cough, for clearing away heat, for promoting the flow of qi, for dispelling dampness, or tonics, should be added to them in line with the different accompanying symptoms and the patient's constitution.

Peppermint

ORIGIN The branch and leaf of Mentha haplcalyx Briq., family Labiatae.

NATURE, TASTE AND CHANNEL TROPISM Acrid in taste, cool in nature, and attributive to liver and lung channels.

EFFICIENCIES 1. Expel wind and heat, clear away heat from head and eyes and ease the throat.

2. Disperse wind, let out the skin eruption and alleviate itching.

INDICATIONS 1. For common cold of wind—heat type and early stage of seasonal febrile disease with mild chilliness, anhidrosis, headache and general aching, and headache of wind—heat type, eye pain, sore throat.

2. For the early stage of eruptive diseases and urticaria,

DIRECTIONS Decoction: 2—10g (decocted later).

Mulberry Leaf

ORIGIN Leaf of Morus alba L, family Moraceae.

NATURE, TASTE AND CHANNEL TROPISM Bitter and sweet in taste, cold in nature, and attributive to lung and liver channels.

EFFICIENCIES Expel wind and heat, open the depressed lung energy and relieve cough, clear away liver—fire to treat eye disease, cool the blood and stop bleeding, relieve night sweating.

INDICATIONS 1. For common cold and cough of wind—heat type, sorethroat.

2. For wind—heat and liver—fire syndrome with redness, swelling and pain of the eye; for blurring of vision due to hypofunction of liver.

3. For hematemesis and hemoptysis of blood—heat type.

DIRECTIONS Decoction: 3—10g. Powder: 6—9g for night sweat, taken with rice water.

Chrysanthemum Flower

ORIGIN Capitulum of Chrysanthemum morifolium Ramat, family Compositae.

NATURE, TASTE AND CHANNEL TROPISM Acrid, sweet and bitter in taste, slightly cold in nature, and attributive to liver and lung channels.

EFFICIENCIES Expel wind and clear away heat, clear away liver—fire to treat eye disease, calm the sthenic liver energy, clear away heat and toxic materials.

INDICATIONS 1. For common cold of wind—heat type and the early stage of seasonal febrile disease with superficies syndrome.

2. For liver—fire syndrome with redness, swelling and pain of the eye.

3. For headache and dizziness due to hypoactivity of liver—yang.

4. For carbuncle due to intensive heat, usually used with Flos Chrysanthemi Indici.

DIRECTION Decoction: 3—10g; 10—30g for severe heat cases.

Perilla Leaf

ORIGIN The leaf of Perilla frutescens (L.) Britt. var. acuta (Thunb.) Kudo, Family Labiatae.

NATURE, TASTE AND CHANNEL TROPISM Acrid in taste, warm in nature, and attributive to lung and spleen channels.

EFFICIENCIES Induce sweating to expel the exogenous cold evils from the body surface, open inhibited lung energy to relieve cough, promote vital energy circulation and soothe the middle—jiao, relieve fish and crab poisoning.

INDICATIONS 1. For common cold of wind—cold type; cough of wind—cold type with thin sputum and feeling of oppression in the chest; stuffy nose and sneezing due to wind—cold.

2. For nausea and vomiting and morning sickness due to stagnation of spleen—energy and stomach—energy.

3. For abdominal pain, nausea, vomiting and diarrhea after intake of fish and crab. Leaves cooked with fish and crab may prevent the poisoning or allergy.

DLRECTION Decoction: 3—10g.

Fresh Ginger

ORIGIN The fresh rhizome of Zingiber officinale (Willd.) Rosc, family Zingiberaceae.

NATURE, TASTE AND CHANNEL TROPISM Acrid in taste, slightly warm in nature, and attributive to lung and spleen channels.

EFFICIENCIES Induce sweating to expel the exogenous evils from the body surface, warm the lung to relieve cough, warm the middle—jiao to stop vomiting, detoxication.

INDICATIONS 1. For common cold of wind—cold type.

2. For cough of wind—cold type.

3. For vomiting and abdominal pain due to stomach—cold, vomiting due to stomach—heat.

4. For poisoning of fish, crab, Rhizoma Pinelliae and Rhizoma Arisaematis. For preventing the poisoning of the materials mentioned above, Zingiberis Recens should be cooked with fish and crab, and prepared together with Pinelliae and Arisaematis.

DIRECTIONS Decoction: 3—10g.

Elsholtzia

ORIGIN Herb of Elsholtzia splendens Nakai ex F. Maekawa and Mosla chinensis Maxim., family Labiatae.

NATURE, TASTE AND CHANNEL TROPISM Acrid in taste, slightly warm in nature, and attributive to lung and stomach channels.

EFFICIENCIES Induce sweating to expel exogenous evils from the body surface, expel summer—heat and eliminate dampness, promote diuresis and relieve edema.

INDICATIONS 1. For common cold in summer time and summer heat—

dampness syndrome with chilliness, fever, headache and anhidrosis, or vomiting, diarrhea and abdominal pain.

2. For cases of edema and dysuria.

DIRECTIONS　Decoction: 3—10g.

Prepared soybean

ORIGIN　The fermented seeds of Glycine max(L.)Merr., family Leguminosae.

NATURE, TASTE AND CHANNEL TROPISM　Acrid, sweet and slightly bitter in taste, cold in nature, and attributive to lung and stomach channels.

EFFICIENCIES　Expel the exogenous evils from the body surface, get rid of vexation.

INDICATIONS　1. For common cold of wind—heat type, used together with Flos Lonicerae, Herba Menthae, etc.; and with Bulbus Allii Fistulosi for wind—cold type.

2. For later stage of febrile diseases with chest upset and restlessness.

DIRECTIONS　Decoction: 10—15g.

Green Chinese Onion

ORIGIN　Bulb of Allium fistulosum L., family Liliaceae.

NATURE, TASTE AND CHANNEL TROPISM　Acrid in taste, warm in nature, and attributive to lung and stomach channels.

EFFICIENCIES　Induce sweating to expel exogenous evils from the body surface, expel cold and activate yang.

INDICATIONS　1. For common cold of wind—cold type.

2. For false heat—syndrome in appearance but real cold—syndrome in nature, also for abdominal distension and pain due to stagnation of vital energy and cold evil, and for dysuria due to hypofunction of urinary bladder. Fried Allii Fistulosi should be applied over the umbilicus and urinary bladder.

DIRECTION　Decoction: 3—10g.

Coriander

ORIGIN The whole grass with root of Coriandrum sativum, family Umblliferae.

NATURE, TASTE AND CHANNEL TROPISM Pungent in taste, warm in nature, and attributive to lung and spleen channels.

EFFICIENCIES Inducing diaphoresis and promoting eruption, promoting digestion and keeping adverse qi flowing downward.

INDICATIONS It is used to treat slow eruption of measles and food retention.

DIRECTIONS To be eaten after quick—boiled in boiling water, stir—fried, or to be decocted for oral administration or external bathing. It should be avoided by those who suffer from measles that either has erupted or not erupted with toxic heat congested other than attack of wind—cold on body surface.

Section 2

Heat—clearing Drugs

The kind of drugs whose principal action is clearing away the internal heat belongs to the category of dietetic Chinese drugs for heat—clearing.

Most drugs in this class are cool or cold in nature, with the effects of clearing away heat, purging fire, removing heat from the blood, detoxicating, and clearing away heat of the deficiency type. They are chiefly indicated for febrile diseases with high fever, dysentery of heat type, suppurative infections on the body surface and various interior heat—syndromes such as interior heat—syndrome due to yin deficiency. They should be chosen in accordance with different syndromes. For interior heat—syndrome associated with exterior syndrome, drugs for relieving exterior syndrome should be first used, or drugs for relieving exterior as well as interior syndromes should be given simultaneously. When there is pathogenic heat in the qi system accompanied with heat in the blood system, drugs for clearing away heat in both systems should be used.

Honeysuckle Flower

ORIGIN The flower bud of Lonicera japonica Thunb., L. hypoglauca Miq. and L. confusa DC., family Caprifoliaceae.

NATURE, TASTE AND CHANNEL TROPISM Sweet in taste, cold in nature, and attributive to lung, stomach and large intestine channels.

EFFICIENCIES Clear away heat and toxic material, expel wind and heat.

INDICATIONS 1. For the onset of seasonal febrile diseases or exogenous wind—heat syndrome with high fever and mild chilliness, thirst and floating pulse.

2. For qifen sthenia—heat syndrome with high fever, excessive thirst, yellow fur, full and large pulse.

3. For yingfen and xuefen heat syndrome with fever, restlessness and insomnia, skin eruption, crimson and dry tongue.

4. For sorethroat, skin infections.

5. For dysentery due to intense heat—toxic.

DIRECTION Decoction: 9—15g, up to 30—60g.

Capejasmine Fruit

ORIGIN Fruit of Gardenia jasminoides Ellis var. radicans (Thunb.) Makino, family Rubiaceae.

NATURE, TASTE AND CHANNEL TROPISM Bitter in taste, cold in nature, and attributive to liver, lung, stomach and triple—jiao channels.

EFFICIENCIES Purge sthenic fire to relieve vexation, clear away heat and promote diuresis, clear away heat and toxic materials, cool the blood and stop bleeding, remove blood stasis and alleviate pain.

INDICATIONS 1. For febrile diseases with irritability, insomnia, and even high fever, coma and delirium.

2. For jaundice and stranguria of dampness—heat type.

3. For skin infection of intense heat type, erysipelas, burn and conjunctivitis.

4. For heat—syndrome with hematemesis, hemoptysis, epistaxis, hematuria, hemafecia, metrorrhagia, etc.

5. For trauma with local swelling and pain (external use).

DIRECTIONS Decoction: 3—9g. External use: Appropriate amount.

Patrinin

ORIGIN Herb of Patrinia villosa Juss. or P. scabiosaefolia Fisch., family Valerianaceae.

NATURE, TASTE AND CHANNEL TROPISM Acrid and bitter in taste, cool in nature, and attributive to stomach, large intestine and liver channels.

EFFICIENCIES Remove blood stasis and alleviate pain, clear away heat and toxic material, relieve abscess and promote pus drainage and tranquilizing.

INDICATIONS 1. For acute appendicitis, pulmonary abscess and skin infection. Recently also for pancreatitis, tonsillitis; P. vilosa also used for influenza, while P. scabiosaefolia for snake bite.

2. For postpartum abdominal pain and menorrhagia due to blood stasis, chest pain, etc.

3. For vexation, insomnia, insanity.

DIRECTIONS Decoction: 9—30g up to 30—90g for single dose.

Wild Chrysanthemum Flower

ORIGIN The capitulum of Chrysanthemum indicum L., family Compositae.

NATURE, TASTE AND CHANNEL TROPISM Bitter in taste, slightly cold in nature, and attributive to lung and liver channels.

EFFICIENCIES Clear away heat and toxic material, clear away liver—fire.

INDICATIONS 1. For carbuncle, skin nodules, scrofula and sorethroat, also for influenza.

2. For liver—fire syndrome with eye congestion, photophobia and lacrimation and hypertension with headache, irritability, and flushed face, wiry and rapid pulse.

DIRECTION Decoction: 9—15g.

Purslane

ORIGIN Herb of portulaca oleracea L., family portulacaceae.

NATURE, TASTE AND CHANNEL TROPISM Sour in taste, cold in nature, and attributive to large intestine and liver channels.

EFFICIENCIES Clear away heat and toxic material, expel dampness and alleviate itching, alleviate uterine bleeding.

INDICATIONS 1. For diarrhea, dysentery and leucorrhagia of dampness—heat type, hemorrhoids, carbuncle, etc.

2. For eczema, dermatitis, herpes zoster, flat wart, vitiligo, etc.

3. For metrorrhagia and menorrhea.

DIRECTIONS Decoction: 30—60g; appropriate amount for external use.

Cassia Seed

ORIGIN Seed of Cassia obtusifolia L. or C. tora L., family Leguminosae.

NATURE, TASTE AND CHANNEL TROPISM Bitter in taste, slightly cold in nature, and attributive to liver and large intestine channels.

EFFICIENCIES Clear away liver—fire and improve visual acuity, suppress liver—yang, lower blood—fat, relax the bowels.

INDICATIONS 1. For liver—heat or wind—heat syndrome with redness, swelling and pain of the eye, photophobia and lacrimation.

2. For hyperactivity of liver—yang or liver—fire with headache, dizziness, restlessness and bad temper. Recently used for hypertension.

3. For hypercholesterinemia, hypertriglyceridemia and atherosclerosis.

4. For constipation due to accumulation of heat or dryness of the intestine.

DIRECTIONS Decoction: Generally 9—15g, crushed before decocting, 40—50g for lowering blood—fat.

Lotus Plumule

ORIGIN The plumule or young leaf of Nelumbo nucifera Gaertn, family Nymphaeaceae.

NATURE, TASTE AND CHANNEL TROPISM Bitter in taste, cold in nature, and attributive to heart and kidney channels.

EFFICIENCIES Clear away heart—fire and relieve vexation.

INDICATIONS Hyperactivity of heart—fire manifested high fever, restlessness, coma, delirium, and insomnia, or hypertension with such manifestations.

DIRECTIONS Decoction: 1. 5—6. 0g.

Lotus Leaf

ORIGIN The leaf of Nelumbo nucifera Gaertn, family Nymphaeaceae.

NATURE, TASTE AND CHANNEL TROPISM Slightly bitter in taste, mild in nature, and attributive to liver and spleen channels.

EFFICIENCIES Clear away summer—heat, promote the production of body fluid to quench thirst, life up lucid—yang, disperse blood stasis and stop bleeding, reduce the level of blood—fat.

INDICATIONS 1. For summer — heat syndrome with thirst and headache, and diarrhea of summer heat—dampness type.

2. For diarrhea due to spleen—deficiency, used together with Rhizoma Atractylodis Macrocephalae and Rhizoma Dioscoreae.

3. For hematemesis, epistaxis, hemoptysis, hematuria, metrorrhagia, etc.

4. For hypercholesterolemia, hypertriglyceridemia and angina pectoris.

DIRECTIONS Decoction: 6—12g. For reducing blood—fat: 50—150g.

Watermelon Peel

ORIGIN The exocarp of Citrullus lanatus (Thunb.) Mansfeld, family Cucurbitaceae.

NATURE, TASTE AND CHANNEL TROPISM　Sweet and bland in taste, cool in nature, and attributive to spleen and stomach channels.

EFFICIENCIES　Clear away summer — heat, promote the production of fluid and diuresis.

INDICATIONS　For summer—heat syndrome with fever, thirst and oliguria with yellowish urine and edema.

DIRECTION　Decoction: 15—30g.

Mung Bean

ORIGIN The seed of Phaseolus radiatus, family Leguminosae.

NATURE, TASTE AND CHANNEL TROPISM　Sweet in taste, cold in nature, and attributive to heart and lung channels.

EFFICIENCIES　Clear away heat and toxic materials, clear away summer—heat and promote diuresis, relieve the metallic and drug poisoning, external use for clearing away heat and promoting tissue regeneration, reduce the level of blood—fat.

INDICATIONS　1. For preventing and treating summer—heat syndrome and miliaria, and for diarrhea of summer heat — dampness type, carbuncle, mumps, acne, edema and erysipelas.

2. For preventing and treating the poisoning of lead, arsenic, alcohol and Radix Aconiti.

3. For unhealing ruptured carbuncle and furuncle, skin ulcer.

4. For hyperlipemia, hypercholesterolemia, hypertriglyceridemia, hyperlipoproteinemia, etc.

DIRECTION　Decoction: 20—60g up to 100—250g. External use: Appropriate amount.

Towel Gourd

ORIGIN　The fresh tender fruit or Luffa cylindrica of L. acutangula, family Cucurbitaceae.

NATURE, TASTE AND CHANNEL TROPISM　Sweet in flavor and

cool in nature, acting on the channels of the liver and stomach.

EFFICIENCIES Clearing away pathogenic heat and resolve phlegm, cooling the blood and removing toxic materials.

INDICATIONS It is used to treat fever, restlessness and thirst during the course of febrile diseases, dyspnea and cough due to phlegm retention, fresh blood in stools and anal fistula, metrorrhagia and profuse leukorrhea, stranguria with blood, furuncle, galactostasis, carbuncle and swelling.

DIRECTIONS To be eaten cooked, or decocted for oral administration, or pounded to get its juice for application to the affected part. Those who suffer from debility with endogenous cold should not eat it excessively.

Frog

ORIGIN The flesh of Rana nigromaculata or R. plancyi, family Ranidae.

NATURE, TASTE AND CHANNEL TROPISM Sweet in flavor and cool in nature, acting on the channels of the urinary bladder, intestines and stomach.

EFFICIENCIES Clearing away heat and toxic materials, treating deficiency syndrome, inducing diuresis and reducing edema.

INDICATIONS It is used to treat consumptive fever, general edema, malnutrition of children due to impairment of the spleen and stomach, hydrops, dysphagia, dysentery, herpes simplex of children.

DIRECTIONS To be decocted, eaten boiled or stir—fried. It can be used as an ingredient of boluses, pills or powder, or mashed for external application.

Crab

ORIGIN The meat and the internal organs of Eriocheir sinensis, family Grapsidae.

NATURE, TASTE AND CHANNEL TROPISM Salty in taste and cold in nature, acting on the channels of the liver and stomach.

EFFICIENCIES Clearing away heat, removing blood stasis, promoting reunion of fractured bones.

INDICATIONS It is used to treat impairment of muscles and bones, scabies, paint dermatitis and scald.

DIRECTIONS To be eaten boiled, steamed; or to be burned into charcoal and ground into powder for oral administration, or made into boluses or pills for internal use. When used externally, it is to be mashed or dried over a fire and pounded into powder and applied to the affected part after being mixed with water. Precaution should be taken by patients who manifest the symptoms of exterior syndrome, or deficiency—cold of the spleen and stomach or chronic diseases due to pathogenic wind. Being easy to go bad, crabs should be eaten fresh.

Lotus Root

ORIGIN The fat rhizome of Nelumbo nucifera, family Nymphaeaceae.

NATURE, TASTE AND CHANNEL TROPISM Sweet in taste, cold in nature, and attributive to heart, spleen and stomach channels.

EFFICIENCIES 1. Raw lotus root can clear away heat, cool the blood, dissipate blood stasis.

2. Lotus root cooked can strengthen the spleen, promote the functional activity of stomach, replenish the blood, promote the tissue regeneration and arrest diarrhea.

INDICATIONS Raw lotus root is used to treat restlessness and thirst during the course of febrile diseases, hematemesis, nose—bleeding and strangury of heat type.

DIRECTIONS To be eaten raw, cooked, or pounded to get its juice for drinking. It can be dried in the sun and ground into powder for making gruel.

SUPPLEMENT Lotus Root Joint: Its decoction, when taken orally, can check upward adverse flow of qi and regulate the middle—jiao; while its parched charcoal, being able to arrest bleeding and dissipate blood stasis, is used to treat bleeding diseases of various kinds.

Section 3

Purgative Drugs

This kind of drugs which can induce diarrhea and promote laxation of the bowels belongs to the category of purgative drugs of dietetic Chinese drugs.

Most drugs in this class are mild, and they have the effects of relaxing the bowels, clearing away heat, purging fire, dispelling retained fluid and reducing edema. They are indicated for interior syndromes of excess type marked by dry stool, constipation, food stagnation, accumulation of heat of excess type in the interior, edema and fluid retention, but they do not have the disadvantage of causing impairment of the health energy.

Hemp Fruit

ORIGIN The fruit of Cannabis sativa L., family Moraceae.

NATURE, TASTE AND CHANNEL TROPISM Sweet in taste, mild in nature, and attributive to spleen, stomach and large intestine channels.

EFFICIENCIES Moisturize the intestine and relax the bowels, nourish yin and restore vital energy.

INDICATIONS For constipation due to consumption of fluid and dryness of intestine; indicated for febrile disease with consumption of yin and fire hyperactivity, or yin—deficiency, consumption of fluid in the aged, as well as postpartum anemia, also for habitual constipation.

DIRECTIONS Decoction: 9—30g (crushed before decocting).

Bush—cherry Seed

ORIGIN The seed of prunus humilis Bunge or P. japonica Thunb., family Rosaceae.

NATURE, TASTE AND CHANNEL TROPISM Acrid, bitter and sweet in taste, mild in nature, and attributive to large and small intestine channels.

EFFICIENCIES Moisturize the intestine and relax the bowels, promote diuresis and relieve edema.

INDICATIONS 1. For constipation due to stagnation of large intestine or dryness of intestine, habitual constipation, etc.

2. For edema, dysuria and beriberi.

DIRECTIONS Decoction: 6—12g(crushed before decocting).

Honey

ORIGIN The honey made by bees(Apis cerana Fabricius and A. mellifera L., family Apidae). Mainly containing glucose and fructose and small amount of pollen.

NATURE, TASTE AND CHANNEL TROPISM Sweet in taste, mild in nature, and attributive to lung, spleen and large intestine channels.

EFFICIENCIES Nourish the body, moisturize the intestine and relax the bowels, nourish the lung and relieve cough, nourish and strengthen the middle—jiao, alleviate pain, detoxify poisonous effects.

INDICATIONS 1. Oral use or as suppository for constipation occurring in the aged and the puerperants, during convalescence, and those with damage of yin and dryness of intestine.

2. For dry cough, chronic cough due to asthenia of viscera, hemoptysis and sore throat.

3. For abdominal pain due to spleen—deficiency, hypochondriac pain due to liver—deficiency. Recently, used as adjuvant for peptic ulcer, chronic hepatitis, heart disease and neurasthenia attributive to deficiency—syndrome.

4. External use for skin infection, burn and skin ulcer. Also for counteracting the toxicity of Radix Aconiti and Radix Aconiti Praeparata.

DIRECTIONS Oral use: 15—30g.

Section 4

Interior—warming Drugs

This kind of drugs which can warm and dispel internal cold to treat interior cold syndromes are referred to as interior—warming drugs of dietetic Chinese drugs.

Drugs of this class are acrid and hot in nature and can disperse the cold in the interior to normalize the yang—qi or functional activity of the body. These drugs are indicated for gastric and abdominal cold pain, vomiting and diarrhea due to the attack of exogenous cold on the interior and spleen—yang, or for aversion to cold, cold limbs, pale complexion, clear and long urination, pale tongue and thready pulse due to deficiency of yang—qi accompanied with excessive cold in the interior. Some of these drugs have the function of recuperating depleted yang and rescuing the patient from collapse, and therefore they are indicated for yang depletion syndrome.

Interior—warming drugs should be dispensed together with other types of drugs.

Dried Ginger

ORIGIN The rhizome of Zingiber officinale (Willd) Rosc., family Zingiberaceae.

NATURE, TASTE AND CHANNEL TROPISM Acrid in taste, hot in nature, and attributive to heart, lung, spleen and stomach channels.

EFFICIENCIES Dispel cold and warm the middle—jiao, recuperate the depleted yang and dredge the channels, warm the lung and eliminate sputum.

INDICATIONS 1. For deficiency—cold of the middle—jiao with cold pain in the lower abdomen, and diarrhea of cold type, vomiting.

2. For yang—exhaustion syndrome.

3. For phlegm—retention syndrome of lung—cold type with cough and thin

expectoration.

DIRECTIONS Decoction: 3—10g.

Cassia Bark

ORIGIN Bark of Cinnamomum cassia, family Lauraceae.

NATURE, TASTE AND CHANNEL TROPISM Acrid and sweet in taste, extremely heat in nature, and attributive to kidney, spleen, heart and liver channels.

EFFICIENCIES Warm and invigorate spleen—yang and kidney—yang, expel cold and alleviate pain, promote the circulation of vital energy and blood.

INDICATIONS 1. For insufficiency of kidney—yang with soreness and coldness of the loins and legs, impotence, emission, enuresis or frequent micturition, dysuria and edema; for inspiration failure due to kidney hypofunction with dyspnea; for deficiency of spleen—yang and kidney—yang with cold pain of the abdomen, poor appetite, loose stools, or lienteric diarrhea; for flaming—up of deficiency-fire with toothache.

2. For lumbago of cold-dampness type, colic of cold type dysmenorrhea and precordial pain due to stagnation of cold.

3. For insufficiency of vital energy and blood.

DIRECTION Decoction: 1—3g, prepared as powder or thin pieces before decocting, only cooked for a short time. Powder or Pill: 1. 0—1. 5g.

Pricklyash Peel

ORIGIN The peel of Zanthoxylum bungeanum Maxim. or Z. Schinifolium Sieb. et Zucc., family Rutaceae.

NATURE, TASTE AND CHANNEL TROPISM Acrid in taste, warm in nature, and attributive to spleen, stomach and kidney channels.

EFFICIENCIES Warm the middle jiao to alleviate pain and increase appetite, kill parasites, and be lactifuge.

INDICATIONS 1. For deficiency—cold of spleen and stomach with epigastric and abdominal cold pain, vomiting, diarrhea and poor appetite.

2. For roundworm infection with abdominal pain or deficiency—cold syndrome of spleen and stomach; also for schistosomiasis and oxyuriasis.

3. For galactostasis.

DIRECTION Decoction: 2—5g; 6—15g daily for lactifuge.

Retention enema: 4—5% decoction 25—30 ml for 3—4 nights successively for oxyuriasis.

Cloves

ORIGIN The flower bud of Eugenia caryophyllata Thunb., family Myrtaceae.

NATURE, TASTE AND CHANNEL TROPISM Acrid in taste, warm in nature, and attributive to spleen, stomach and kidney channels.

EFFICIENCIES Warm the middle jiao and lower the adverse rising energy, warm the kidney and strengthen yang.

INDICATIONS 1. For stomach—cold syndrome with vomiting, hiccup, poor appetite and loose stool.

2. For impotence due to yang deficiency.

DIRECTION Decoction: 2—5g.

Galangal Rhizome

ORIGIN The rhizome of Alpinia officinarum Hance, family Zingiberaceae.

NATURE, TASTE AND CHANNEL TROPISM Acrid in taste, heat in nature, and attributive to spleen and stomach channels.

EFFICIENCIES Dispel cold, warm the middle jiao, alleviate pain and relieve vomiting.

INDICATIONS For deficiency—cold of the middle jiao with cold pain in the abdomen and vomiting.

DIRECTIONS Decoction: 3—10g.

Aniseed

ORIGIN The fruit of Foeniculum vulgare Mill., family Umbelliferae.

NATURE, TASTE AND CHANNEL TROPISM Acrid in taste, warm in nature, and attributive to liver, kidney, spleen and stomach channels.

EFFICIENCIES Expel cold and alleviate pain, disperse the depressed liver energy and regulate the stomach energy.

INDICATIONS For colic of cold type and orchidoptosis. Recently, used for inguinal hernia, swelling of epididymis, hydrocele testis; also for stomach—cold syndrome with cold pain, and fullness in the epigastrium and abdomen, vomiting and poor appetite.

DIRECTIONS Decoction: 3—9g.

Pepper

ORIGIN The fruit of Piper nigrum L., family Piperaceae.

NATRUE, TASTE AND CHANNEL TROPISM Acrid in taste, heat in nature, and attributive to stomach and large intestine channels.

EFFICIENCIES Warm the middle—jiao to increase appetite, eliminate phlegm.

INDICATIONS 1. For stomach—cold syndrome with abdominal pain, vomiting, diarrhea and anorexia.

2. For deficiency—cold of lung and spleen with cough and thin expectoration, also for epilepsy.

DIRECTIONS Decoction: 2—4g crushed before decocting. Powder: 0.5—1.0g once to twice daily.

Alcoholic Drinks

ORIGIN A drink made from any of rice, wheat, millet, broom millet, Chinese sorghum and others with leaven.

NATURE, TASTE AND CHANNEL TROPISM Bitter, sweet and acrid in taste, warm and toxic in nature, and attributive to heart, liver, lung and stomach channels.

EFFICIENCIES Promoting blood circulation, preventing pathogenic cold, enlivening the spleen, warming the middle—jiao and helping drugs to take effect soon.

INDICATIONS It is used to treat arthralgia due to wind—cold, spasm of muscles, obstruction of qi in the chest, cold sensation and pain in the chest and abdomen.

DIRECTIONS Take it warm together with rice or bread; decoct it along with Chinese drugs or soak Chinese drugs in it for oral administration. It can also be used for drip — bathing, mouth — rinsing, or spread on the affected part. It sholud be avoided by those who indicate syndrome of deficiency of yin, loss of blood or excessive damp—heat.

Section 5

Aromatic Drugs for Resolving Dampness

The kind of drugs which have an aromatic character and the ability to invigorate the spleen and resolve dampness, belongs to the category of aromatic drugs for resolving dampness of dietetic Chinese drugs.

They have a acrid flavour and warm property with an aroma. They have the actions of regulating the functional activities of qi, promoting the elimination of pathogenic dampness, invigorating the spleen and strengthening the stomach. These drugs are suitable for disturbance of the middle — jiao due to dampness marked by epigastric dullness, abdominal distension, nausea and acid regurgitation, loose stool, anorexia, lassitude, sweet taste in the mouth, excessive salivation, whitish greasy coating on the tongue, etc.

Any of these drugs should be used in combination with other types of drugs according to the different types of pathogenic dampness: for cold—dampness, it is used together with drugs for warming the interior; for damp — heat, it is used with drugs for eliminating heat and dampness.

Agastache

ORIGIN The branch and leaf of Pogostemon cablin (Blanco)Benth. ,family Labiatae.

NATURE,TASTE AND CHANNEL TROPISM Acrid in taste,slightly warm in nature,and attributive to spleen,stomach and lung channels.

EFFICIENCIES Eliminate dampness from the middle jiao, regulate the middle jiao and stop vomiting,eliminate summer—heat and expel the affection of exogenous summer—heat and dampness.

INDICATIONS 1. For dampness — syndrome involving the spleen with fullness of the chest and epigastrium,anorexia and greasy feeling in the mouth, for summer — heat dampness syndrome and summer — heat febrile disease,used together with drugs for expelling dampness also for thrush,mycotic enteritis and vaginitis.

2. For dampness — retention syndrome with nausea, vomiting, abdominal pain,diarrhea and morning sickness.

3. For affection of exogenous wind—cold with retention of dampness in the interior manifested as chilliness, fever, heaviness and pain of the head and the body,fullness of the chest,nausea,etc.

DIRECTION Decoction: 3 — 10g, (decocted later); 30 — 60g both orally and topically for thrush and mycotic vaginitis.

Amomum Fruit

ORIGIN The fruit of Amomum villosum Lour. or A. longiligulare T. L. Wu,family Zingiberaceae.

NATURE,TASTE AND CHANNEL TROPISM Acrid in taste,warm in natrue,and attributive to spleen,stomach and kidney channels.

EFFICIENCIES Eliminate dampness and promote the circulation of vital energy,strengthen the stomach and stop vomiting,prevent miscarriage.

INDICATIONS 1. For dampness—syndrome involving spleen—yang and stagnation of spleen energy and stomach energy with feeling of fullness and distending pain in the chest and upper abdomen and loss of appetite;for deficiency—cold of spleen and stomach or dampness—stagnation syndrome with nausea,vomiting, diarrhea and abdominal pain.

2. For threatened abortion due to stagnation of vital energy.

DIRECTION Decoction: 3—10g (decocted later).

Hyacinth Flower

ORIGIN The primary flower of Dolichos lablab L., family Leguminosae.

NATURE, TASTE AND CHANNEL TROPISM Sweet in taste, mild in nature, and attributive to spleen and stomach channels.

EFFICIENCIES Clear away summer—heat and eliminate dampness from the upper—jiao, invigorate the spleen and strengthen the stomach.

INDICATIONS For summer heat—dampness syndrome with feeling of oppression in the chest, dysuria and diarrhea, vomiting, diarrhea and dysentery of dampness—heat type, leucorrhagia, especially suitable for those with dampness—heat in the spleen.

DIRECTION Decoction: 3—9g

Section 6

Drugs for Regulating Qi

This kind of drugs whose principal action is regulating the functional activities of vital energy and enabling the vital energy to circulate normally belongs to the category of dietetic Chinese drugs for regulating qi.

This class of most drugs have a fragrant and warm nature with acrid and bitter in taste. They have the effects of promoting the circulating of vital energy to relieve pain, regulating the activities of vital energy to check the disorder of vital energy, or removing stagnation of vital energy to dissolve mass. They are indicated for stagnation of vital energy and reversed circulation of vital energy due to disorder of the functional activities of vital energy.

Drugs of this class can be selected for use together with other types of drug with regard to different syndromes.

Tangerine Peel

ORIGIN The pericarp of Citrus reticulata Blanco, family Rutaceae.

NATURE, TASTE AND CHANNEL TROPISM Bitter and acrid in taste, warm in nature, and attributive to spleen and lung channels.

EFFICIENCIES Activate vital energy circulation and invigorate spleen, deprive dampness and eliminate phlegm, lower the adverse rising energy and stop vomiting, relieve local infection.

INDICATIONS 1. For stomach—cold and stagnation of vital energy with fullness and pain in the abdomen and vomiting.

2. For spleen—deficiency and stagnation of vital energy with poor appetite, loose stool, fullness of the abdomen.

3. For dampness—retention syndrome involving spleen—yang with fullness of the abdomen, nausea, vomiting, fatigue, poor appetite and loose stool.

4. For phlegm—dampness syndrome with productive cough and thin expectoration. For vomiting due to stomach—cold, for that due to deficiency—cold of spleen and stomach, for that due to stomach—heat.

5. For carbuncle, especially for acute mastitis.

DIRECTION Decoction: 3—9g; 30—40g for relieving local infection.

Green Tangerine Peel

ORIGIN The immature fruit or its pericarp of Citrus reticulata Blanco, family Rutaceae.

NATURE, TASTE AND CHANNEL TROPISM Bitter and acrid in taste, warm in nature, and attributive to liver, gallbladder and stomach channels.

EFFICIENCIES Activate vital energy circulation, disperse the stagnated liver energy and alleviate pain, promote digestion and relieve dyspepsia.

INDICATIONS 1. For stagnation of liver energy with hypochondriac pain, lump and pain of the breast, and swelling and pain of testis.

2. For distension and pain of the epigastrium due to indigestion and gas re-

tention, mass and pain of the hypochondrium and upper abdomen due to stagnation of blood and vital energy. Recently, used for hepatic and biliary diseases and fibrous hyperplasia of breast.

DIRECTIONS Decoction: 3—9g.

Tangerine

ORIGIN The ripe fruit of various kinds of tangerines such as Citrus tangerina or C. erythrosa, family Rutaceae.

NATURE, TASTE AND CHANNEL TROPISM Sweet, sour in taste, cool in nature, and attributive to lung and stomach channels.

EFFICIENCIES Promoting the function of stomach and regulating the flow of qi, relieving thirst and moisturizing the lung.

INDICATIONS It is used to treat accumulation of qi in the chest and diaphragm, vomiting and poor appetite, insufficiency of stomach—yin, dry mouth and thirst, cough due to retention of pathogenic heat in the lung and excessive drinking.

DIRECTIONS Eat it raw after peeling, or sqeeze its juice out for oral administration. Those who have cough caused by wind—cold or phlegm—retention should not take it.

Finger Citron

ORIGIN The fruit of Citrus medica L. var. sarcodactylis Swingly, family Rutaceae.

NATURE, TASTE AND CHANNEL TROPISM Acrid, bitter and sour in taste, warm in nature, and attributive to liver, spleen and lung channels.

EFFICIENCIES Disperse the stagnated liver energy, activate vital energy circulation and alleviate pain. regulate the stomach and strengthen the spleen. activate vital energy circulation and eliminate phlegm.

INDICATIONS 1. For stagnation of liver energy with distension and pain of the hypochondria and breast, dysmenorrhea or irregular menstruation, especially for those with insufficiency of liver—yin.

2. For spleen hypofunction and stagnation of vital energy with pain and fullness of the upper abdomen, and poor appetite.

3. For phlegm—dampness syndrome with productive cough and dyspnea.

DIRECTIONS Decoction: 3—9g.

Macrostem

ORIGIN The bulb of Allium maerostemon Bunge, family Liliaceae.

NATURE, TASTE AND CHANNEL TROPISM Acrid and bitter in taste, warm in nature, and attributive to lung, heart, stomach and large intestine channels.

EFFICIENCIES Activate vital energy circulation and alleviate pain, activate yang and disperse lumps, keep the adverse energy downward and relieve the stagnation of intestines.

INDICATIONS 1. For phlegm—syndrome of cold—dampness type with chest pain, cough and dyspnea.

2. For dysentery with tenesmus.

DIRECTIONS Decoction: 9—15g.

Garlic

ORIGIN The bulb of Allium sativum, family Liliaceae.

NATURE, TASTE AND CHANNEL TROPISM Acrid in taste, warm in nature, and attributive to spleen, stomach and lung channels.

EFFICIENCIES Promoting the circulation of retained qi, warming the spleen and stomach, removing mass in the abdomen, clearing away toxic materials, destroying intestinal worms.

INDICATIONS It is used to treat retention of food in the stomach, cold sensation and pain in the abdomen, hydrops, turgor, diarrhea, dysentery, malaria, whoopy cough, boils and pyogenic infections, tinea capitis and snake bite.

DIRECTIONS To be eaten raw, mashed, or decocted for internal use. It can also be pounded to get its juice for external application to the affected part, or sliced for moxibustion at acupuncture points. Garlic being pungent in flavor and warm in nature, excessive eating will cause heat and irritation to some part of the body, so it should be avoided if one either indicates syndrome of hyperactivity of fire owing to yin deficiency or suffers from diseases in the eye, mouth or tongue.

Buckwheat

ORIGIN The seed of Fagopyrum esculentum, family Polygonaceae.

NATURE, TASTE AND CHANNEL TROPISM Sweet in taste, cool in nature, and attributive to spleen, stomach and large intestine channels.

EFFICIENCIES Promoting functional activity of the stomach and relieving intestine stuffiness, keeping the adverse qi flowing downward and removing food stagnancy, and removing noxious damp—heat.

INDICATIONS It is used to treat summer cholera, retention of food in the stomach and intestines, chronic diarrhea, fasting dysentery, wandering erysi—pelas, lumbodorsal carbuncle, scrofula and scald burn.

DIRECTIONS To be made into thin gruel, or boluses or powder out of its flour for internal use. It can also be ground into powder for external application. It should not be taken for long, and it should be avoided if one suffers from insufficiency of the spleen—yang.

Siberian Filbert

ORIGIN The shelled seed of Corylus heterophylla, family Betulaceae.

NATURE, TASTE AND CHANNEL TROPISM Sweet in taste and neutral in nature, acting on the channels of the stomach and spleen.

EFFICIENCIES Regulating the function of the spleen and stomach, inducing appetite and digestion, improving eyesight.

INDICATIONS It is used for treatment of poor appetite, tiredness, liability to fatigue, dim eyesight, emaciation, etc.

DIRECTIONS To be eaten parched, or ground into powder for oral administration, or decocted along with other Chinese herbs.

Mushroom

ORIGIN The whole substance of Agaricus campestris, family Agarocaceae.

NATURE, TASTE AND CHANNEL TROPISM Sweet in taste, cool in nature, and attributive to intestines, stomach and lung channels.

EFFICIENCIES Promoting the functional activity of stomach, regulating the flow of qi, resolving phlegm, pleasing the mind, clearing away toxic materials, inducing eruption of measles, arresting vomiting and diarrhea.

INDICATIONS It is used to treat febrile diseases at the middle or late stage, bodily tiredness and deficiency of qi, dry mouth and anorexia, cough with phlegm, fullness sensation and oppressed feeling in the chest, vomiting, diarrhea, slow eruption of measles in children. Mushroom can also be used as an auixliary treatment of infectious hepatitis and leukopenia.

DIRECTIONS To be decocted, eat cooked or sauted.

Yellow Soybean

ORIGIN The yellow—skin seed of Glycine max, family Leguminosae.

NATURE, TASTE AND CHANNEL TROPISM Sweet in taste and neutral in nature, acting on the channels of the spleen and large intestine.

EFFICIENCIES Strengthening the spleen and relieving epigastric distention, moistening dryness and inducing diuresis.

INDICATIONS It is used for treatment of infantile malnutrition, diarrhea, dysentery, abdominal distention, emaciation, toxemia of pregnancy, pyogenic infections of skin and external diseases (such as carbuncle, deep—rooted carbuncle, furuncle, multiple abscess, scrofula, ulcer), and bleeding due to injury. Being antibacterial and antiphlogistic, soybean is effective for pharyngitis, conjunctivitis, stomatitis, bacillary dysentery and enteritis.

DIRECTIONS To be made into cooked food, soybean milk for oral administration, or ground into powder for external application. Raw soybean is used for soothing the liver and regulating the circulation of qi, while cooked soybean is used for invigoration.

Section 7

Drugs for Promoting Blood Circulation and Removing Blood Stasis

This kind of drugs whose principal effects are to make free the passage of blood in the vessels, promote blood circulation and disperse blood stasis are termed as drugs for promoting blood circulation and removing blood stasis of the dietetic Chinese drugs.

Most drugs of this class have flavour, warm property and actions of promoting blood circulation and dispersing blood stasis to clear the channels, remove obstruction of qi and blood, reduce swelling and relieve pain. They are effective for various syndromes due to obstruction of blood circulation and retention of blood stasis in the interior, and pain in the chest, hypochondrium and abdomen due to stagnation of qi and blood stasis.

Because blood circulates smoothly only when qi is in normal flow, and blood slows down when qi stagnates, therefore, drugs for promoting blood circulation and eliminating blood stasis are often used along with drugs for promoting the flow of qi to strengthen their effects. Apart from this, other suitable drugs should be added according to the causes and symptoms of diseases.

Peach Kernel

ORIGIN The seed of Prunus persica (L.) Batsch and P. davidiana Franch., family Rosaceae.

NATURE, TASTE AND CHANNEL TROPISM Bitter and sweet in taste, mild in nature, and attributive to lung, liver and large intestine channels.

EFFICIENCIES Promote blood circulation, remove blood stasis and relieve carbuncle, relieve cough and asthma, promote blood circulation and moisturize dryness, moisturize the intestine and relax the bowels.

INDICATIONS 1. For blood — stasis syndrome with anemia, dysmenorrhea and abdominal mass. Recently, used for hysteromyoma. Also for trauma, especially the injury of the chest, abdomen and spine, for acute appendicitis. Recently, injections are used for central retinitis, pigmentary degeneration of retina, postocluar optic neuritis, optic atrophy, etc.

2. For cough and asthma.

3. For blood stasis and blood dryness with pruritic eruptions.

4. For constipation due to dryness of the intestine.

DIRECTIONS Decoction: 6—12g (crushed before decocting). The spermoderm should be retained for asthma.

Injection: 100% solution, 2 ml IM daily for diseases of fundus aculi 1 ml postocular injection every other day, 10 times as 1 course.

Safflower

ORIGIN The flower of Carthamus tinctorius L. , family Compositae.

NATURE, TASTE AND CHANNEL TROPISM Acrid in taste, warm in nature, and attributive to heart and liver channels.

EFFICIENCIES Promote blood circulation to remove blood stasis, promote menstruation and alleviate pain, promote blood circulation to relieve carbuncle, promote blood circulation and let out the skin eruption.

INDICATIONS 1. For blood—stasis syndrome with anemia, dysmenorrhea, or postpartum abdominal pain. Recently, for ischemic apoplexy, angina pectoris, thromboangiitis obliterans, sudden deafness, sclerederma neonatorum, flat wart, neurodermatitis, etc.

2. For preventing and treating bed sore (external use); for conjunctivitis and the early stage of the carbuncle.

3. For blood stasis with impediment of skin eruptions.

DIRECTIONS Decoction: 0. 6—1. 0g for promoting blood production; 2. 0—2. 5g for regulating blood; 3—9g promoting blood circulation; 9—12g for removing blood stasis.

Pangolin Scules

ORIGIN　The scales of Manis pentadactyla L. ,family Mandae. Fried with sand to yellow and expanded by soaking in the water,named as prepared pangolin scales.

NATURE,TASTE AND CHANNEL TROPISM _Salty in taste,cold in nature,and attributive to liver and stomach channels.

EFFICIENCIES　Promote blood circulation to remove blood stasis,disperse lumps,relieve carbuncle,drain pus,and open channels,and lactogenesis.

INDICATIONS　1. For blood－stasis syndrome with anemia,dysmenorrhea,abdominal mass,subcutaneous nodule,scrofula,the early stage of the carbuncle,or unruptured abscess,or chronic rheumatism with pain,spasm and stiffness of extremities.

2. For galactostasis.

DIRECTION　Decoction:3－9g. Powder:1. 0－1. 5g bid or tid.

CAUTION　Should be prepared before use. Contraindicated for pregnant women and menorrhalgia.

Red Sage Root

ORIGIN　The root and rhizome of Salvia miltiorrhiza Bwnge. ,family Labiatae.

NATURE,TASTE AND CHANNEL TROPISM　Bitterin taste,slightly cold in nature,acting on the heart,pericardium and liver channels.

EFFICIENCIES　Invigorating blood circulation,removing blood stasis,cooling the blood ,treating carbuncles,and tranquilizing the disturbed mind by nourishing the blood.

INDICATIONS　1. Various syndromes due to accumulation of blood stasis. Slightly cold in property,it is especially effective for diseases due to blood stasis accompanied with heat in the blood. For Cardiodynia,hypochondriac pain,abdominal pain,stomachache,dysmenorrhea,amenorrhea,lochiorrhea and trauma with blood stasis.

2. For sores,carbuncles and other pyogenic skin infections. It is often used with honeysuckle flower,forsythia fruit,frankincense and myrrh.

3. For Vexation and insomnia due to impairment of ying and yin by

pathogenic heat.

In recent years, it has often been used in treating hepatosplenomegaly, coronary heart disease, thromboangiitis obliterans and ectopic pregnancy, and has shown curatve effects.

DIRECTION 5-15g, decocted in water for an oral dose. For thromboangiitis obliterans and arthritis of heat type, the maximum dosage can be 30-60g. Red sage root stir-baked with wine has a stronger effect for promoting blood circulation and eliminating blood stasis.

Section 8

Hemostatics

This kind of drugs whose principal effects are to stop internal and external bleedings is referred to as hemostatics of dietetic Chinese drugs.

They are indicated for various kinds of hemorrhage, such as hemoptysis, epistaxis, hematemesis, hematuria, hemafecia, metrorrhagia and metrostaxis, purpura and traumatic bleeding.

Fielg Thistle

ORIGIN The aerial parts of Cephalanoplos segetum (Bunge) Kitam., family Compositae.

NATURE, TASTE AND CHANNEL TROPISM Sweet in taste, cool in nature, and attributive to liver and spleen channels.

EFFICIENCIES Cool the blood and stop bleeding, promote diuresis, clear away heat and toxic material.

INDICATIONS 1. Generally for hematuria, metrorrhagia, also for hematemesis, hemoptysis, hemafecia, etc., especially for bleeding due to blood — heat.

2. For jaundice of dampness — heat type, edema and dysuria, recently used

for acute and chronic infectious hepatitis.

3. For skin infection and acute eczema.

DIRECTION Decoction: 10—15g; 20—60g of fresh herb.

Boked Ginger

ORIGIN The dried rhizome of Zingiber officinale (Willd), Rosc., family Zingiberaceae.

NATURE, TASTE AND CHANNEL TROPISM Bitter and acrid in taste, hot in nature, and attributive to spleen and liver channels.

EFFICIENCIES Warm the meridian to stop bleeding, warm the meridian to alleviate pain.

INDICATIONS 1. For hematemesis, hemafecia, hemoptysis and metrorrhagia of asthenia—cold type.

2. For abdominal pain and postpartum abdominal pain of asthenia—cold type.

DIRECTION Decoction: 3—6g. Powder: 1—2g bid or tid.

Sophora Flower

ORIGIN The flower bud of Sophora japonica L., family Leguminosae.

NATURE, TASTE AND CHANNEL TROPISM Bitter in taste, mild in nature, and attributive to stomach, liver and large intestine channels.

EFFICIENCIES Cool the blood and stop bleeding, clear away liver—heat and lower blood pressure.

INDICATIONS 1. Generally used for hemorrhoids, hematemesis and hemafecia, also for hemoptysis, metrorrhagia, etc.

2. For hypertension.

DIRECTIONS Decoction: 9—12g, up to 30—60g.

Shepherd's Purse

ORIGIN Herb of Capsella bursa—pastoris(L.)Medic. ,family Cruciferae.

NATURE, TASTE AND CHANNEL TROPISM Sweet and bland in taste, slightly cool in nature, and attributive to liver, stomach, small intestine and urinary bladder channels.

EFFICIENCIES Cool the blood and stop bleeding, clear away heat and promote diuresis, lower blood pressure.

INDICATIONS 1. Generally for metrorrhagia and hematuria, also for hematemesis, hemoptysis, etc.

2. For stranguria complicated by chyluria, edema and dysuria.

3. For hypertension.

DIRECTION Decoction: 15—30g; 30—60g of fresh herb.

Spinach

ORIGIN The whole grass of Spinacia oleracea, family Chenopodiaceae.

NATURE, TASTE AND CHANNEL TROPISM Sweet in taste and cool in nature, acting on the channels of the large intestine and stomach.

EFFICIENCIES Nourishing the blood, arresting bleeding, astringing yin fluid, moistening dryness.

INDICATIONS It is used as a cure of nose—bleeding, hemafecia, scurvy, polydipsia due to diabetes, difficulty of feces. It has been used recently for treatment of anemia.

DIRECTIONS To be eaten tenderly sauted, cooked, quick—boiled in boiling water, or decocted for oral administration. Those who show symptoms of debility and loose stools should not take it.

Section 9

Antirhumatics

The kind of drugs which can eliminate pathogenic wind and dampness and relieve arthralgia are referred to as antirheumatics of dietetic Chinese drugs.

They are capable of eliminating the pathogenic wind—dampness from the muscles, channels and collaterals, tendons and bones, Some of them have the effects of relaxing the muscles and tendons, clearing and activating the channels and collaterals, relieving pain and strengthening the tendons and bones by nourishing the liver and kidney. These drugs are effective for arthralgia due to wind—dampness, spasm of muscles, numbness and hypoesthesia, hemiplegia, aching loins and knees, flaccidity of the lower limbs and other symptoms.

This kind of suitable drugs should be selected according to the actual conditions such as the characteristics and locations of different types of arthralgia—syndrome, and should be used in combination with other kinds of drugs.

Fruit of Common Flower—ingquince

ORIGIN Fruit of Chaenomeles speciosa (Sweet) Nakai or C. sinensis (Thouin) Koehne, family Rosaceae.

NATURE, TASTE AND CHANNEL TROPISM Sour in taste, warm in nature, and attributive to liver and spleen channels.

EFFICIENCIES Expel wind—dampness, relax the tendons, regulate the stomach and eliminate dampness, promote digestion.

INDICATIONS 1. For arthralgia of wind—dampness type manifested as feeling of heaviness and stiffness of extremities and muscular spasm. Also for beriberi.

2. For vomiting, diarrhea, abdominal pain and muscular spasm of summer—heat and dampness type, for diarrhea of dampness origin.

3. For indigestion.

DIRECTIONS Decoction: 6—12g.

Tiger Bone

ORIGIN The bones of Panthera tigris L. family Felidae.

NATURE, TASTE AND CHANNEL TROPISM Acrid and sweet in taste, warm in nature, and attributive to liver and kidney channels.

EFFICIENCIES Expel wind and alleviate pain, strengthen the bones and muscles.

INDICATIONS For rheumatism and flaccidity of the back and lower extremities caused by deficiency of the cold of the liver and kidney. Recently, its preparation of wine and injection are used for rheumatic arthritis and rheumatoid arthritis.

DIRECTION Decoction: 10—15g.

Black Snake

ORIGIN The whole body (viscera discarded) of Zaocys dhumnades Cantor, family Colubridae.

NATURE, TASTE CHANNEL TROPISM Sweet in taste, mild in nature, mildly toxic, and attributive to liver channel.

EFFICIENCIES Expel wind, dredge the channels, relieve muscular spasm, relieve convulsive seizures, expel wind and alleviate itching, remove toxic materials.

INDICATIONS 1. For rheumatism, especially the intractable cases and those with wandering arthralgia, numbness of the extremities and muscular spasm; also for apoplexy complicated by distortion of face and hemiplegia.

2. For infantile convulsion, tetanus and convulsion after apoplexy.

3. For itching induced by scabies, tinea infection and urticaria.

4. For leprosy, scrofula, and severe skin infections.

DIRECTION Decoction: 3—10g, Powder: 1. 0—1. 5g.

Pine Nut

ORIGIN The seed of Pinus koraiensis, family Pinaceae.

NATURE, TASTE AND CHANNEL TROPISM Sweet in taste and warm in nature, acting on the channels of the liver, lung and large intestine.

EFFICIENCIES Arresting convulsion, moisturizing the lung, lubricating the intestinal tract and promoting the production of body fluid.

INDICATIONS It is used as a cure of migratory arthralgia, vertigo, dry cough, hemoptysis and constipation.

DIRECTIONS To be eaten after parched to such a degree that fragrance is given out, or to be taken decocted as a drink, or used as an ingredient of a medicament. It should be avoided by those who are troubled with loose stools, sperma—torrhoea or phlegm—dampness.

Wild Goose Meat

ORIGIN The meat of Anser albifrons (scopoli), A. cygnoides, etc, family Anatidae.

NATURE, TASTE AND CHANNEL TROPISM Sweet in taste, neutral in nature, and attributive to lung, liver and kidney channels.

EFFICIENCIES Dispersing pathogenic wind, strengthening the bone, tendon and muscle.

INDICATIONS It is used to treat obstinate numbness of the extremities and migratory arthralgia.

DIRECTIONS To be eaten stewed, stir—fried or decocted for drinking.

Section 10

Druga for Inducing Diuresis and Excreting Dampness

The kind of drugs which can clear and regulate water passages and excrete dampness belongs to the category of dietetic Chinese drugs for inducing diuresis and excreting dampness.

These drugs can increase the amount of unine and make micturition easy, and as a result, the water dampness in the body can be excreted out through urination, Some of these drugs also have the effects of eliminating damp—heat. These drugs are indicated for dysuria, edema, stranguria, phlegm retention, damp—warm syndrome, jaundice, exudative wound, etc. Most of drugs of this type are sweet or tasteless in flavour and neutral, slightly cold or cold in nature.

Drugs for inducing diuresis and excreting dampness should be used in combination with other types of drugs according to the conditions.

Job's—tears Seed

ORIGIN The dried matrue seed of Coix lacryma—jobi L. var. ma—yuen (Roman.) Stapf, family Gramineae.

NATURE, TASTE AND CHANNEL TROPISM Sweet and bland in taste, slightly cold in nature, and attributive to spleen, stomach, lung and large intestine channels.

EFFICIENCIES Promote diuresis and invigorate the spleen, relieve dampness obstruction and relax the muscles, clear away heat to drain the pus.

INDICATIONS 1. For spleen—deficiency syndrome with accumulation of dampness manifested as edema, beriberi or diarrhea; for stranguria of dampness—heat type and of stone origin; for dampness febrile disease manifested as fever, bodily heaviness, oppressive sensation over the chest and epigastrium, anorexia, and smooth or greasy tongue coating.

2. For arthralgia of wind—dampness type and muscular rigidity.

3. For lung abscess.

DIRECTIONS Decoction: 10—30g.

Plantain Seed

ORIGIN Seed of Plantago asiatica L. and other species of the same genus, family Plantaginaceae.

NATURE, TASTE AND CHANNEL TROPISM Sweet in taste, cold in nature, and attributive to lung, urinary bladder, small intestine, kidney and liver channels.

EFFICIENCIES Clear away heat, promote diuresis and relieve stranguria, clear away heat to improve visual acuity, eliminate sputum and relieve cough.

INDICATIONS 1. For stranguria of heat type or of urinary stone origin, edema and diarrhea of dampness—heat or summer—heat and dampness type.

2. For conjunctivitis of liver—heat origin; for dim eyesight due to liver—deficiency, used together with liver—nourishing herbs.

3. For cough of lung—heat type.

DIRECTION Decoction: 3—15g (wrapped with cloth for boiling).

Wax Gourd Peel

ORIGIN The exocarpium of Benincasa hispida (Thunb) Cong., family Cucurbitaceae.

NATURE, TASTE AND CHANNEL TROPISM Sweet in taste, slightly cold in nature, and attributive to kidney, stomach and small intestine channels.

EFFICIENCIES Promote diuresis to relieve edema, clear away summer—heat.

INDICATION 1. For edema and dysuria.

2. For summer—heat syndrome with thirst oliguria and reddish urine.

DIRECTION Decoction: 15—30g.

Red Phaseolus Bean

ORIGIN Seed of Phaseolus calcaratus Roxb. or P. angularis Wight, family Leguminosae.

NATURE, TASTE AND CHANNEL TROPISM Sweet and sour in taste, mild in nature, and attributive to spleen, heart and small intestine channels.

EFFICIENCIES Promote diuresis to eliminate dampness, detoxify and promote drainage of pus.

INDICATIONS 1. For edema, ascites, dysuria, wet beriberi, diarrhea and jaundice.

2. For skin infection (both oral and external use available).

DIRECTIONS Decoction: 10—30g. External use: Appropriate amount.

Corn Stigma

ORIGIN The style and stigma of Zea mays L. ,family Gramineae.

NATRUE, TASTE CHANNEL TROPISM Sweet in taste and mild in natrue.

EFFICIENCIES Promote diuresis to relieve edema, promote choleresis and relieve jaundice, lower blood pressure, lower blood sugar level, stop bleeding.

INDICATIONS 1. For edema, ascites, wet beriberi, stranguria of heat type and that caused by urinary stone.

2. For hepatocellular jaundice, cholelithiasis and cholecystitis.

3. For hypertension and diabetes mellitus.

4. For epistaxis, gingival bleeding. Recently, also used for thrombocytopenic purpura.

DIRECTION Decoction: 15—30g.

Carp

ORIGIN The flesh or the whole of Cyprinus carpio, family Cyprinidae.

NATURE, TASTE AND CHANNEL TROPISM Sweet in taste and neutral in nature, acting on the channels of the spleen and kidney.

EFFICIENCIES Inducing diuresis to reduce edema, keeping the adverse qi flowing downward, promoting lactation.

INDICATIONS It is used to treat hydrops with turgor, beriberi, jaundice, cough and reversed flow of qi, and galactostasis.

DIRECTIONS To be prepared in any of the following ways; boiled in clear soup or steamed, sweetened and vinegared, boiled in mellow wine and stewed.

Wax Gourd

ORIGIN The fruit of Benincasa hispida, family Cucurbitaceae.

NATURE, TASTE AND CHANNEL TROPISM Sweet, bland in taste and cool in nature, acting on the channels of the lung, large intestine, small intestine and urinary bladder.

EFFICIENCIES Inducing diuresis, clearing away phlegm, removing pathogenic heat and poisonous quality of any substance.

INDICATIONS It is used to treat hydrops and turgor, beriberi, stranguria, cough and asthma with rale, fidgets due to summer—heat, diabetes, diarrhea, dysentery, carbuncle and swelling. It can remove fish toxin and alcohol toxin.

DIRECTIONS To be decocted, or eaten stewed, or made into medicated diet, or pounded to get its juice for drinking; raw wax gourd can be applied to the affected part. Cool—natured, it should not be eaten raw, and it should be avoided if a patient suffers from weakness of the spleen and stomach, cold of insufficiency type in the kidney, or lingering diarrhea resulting from a longstanding case.

Crucian Carp

ORIGIN The flesh or the whole substance of Carassius auratus, family Cyprinidae.

NATURE, TASTE AND CHANNEL TROPISM Sweet in taste and neutral in nature, acting on the channels of the spleen, stomach and large intestine.

EFFICIENCIES Strengthening the spleen and inducing diuresis.

INDICATIONS It is used for treatment of the weakness of the spleen and stomach, poor appetite, asthenia, dysentery, hemafecia, hydrops, stranguria, carbuncle and swell—ing, and ulcer.

DIRECTIONS To be boiled in clear soup or steamed, fried, made into medicated diet, used as an ingredient of boluses, pills or powder, It can be pounded for external application.

Chinese Sorghum

ORIGIN The shelled seed of Sorghum vulgare, family Gramineae.

NATURE, TASTE AND CHANNEL TROPISM Sweet in taste and warm in nature, acting on the channels of the spleen and stomach.

EFFICIENCIES Warming the middle—jiao to strengthen the spleen, excreting dampness and arresting dysentery.

INDICATIONS It is used to treat fluid retention due to hypofunction of the spleen, maldigestion, dysentery and difficulty in urination resulting from damp—heat.

DIRECTIONS To be decocted, or to be ground to make cooked food for oral administration, or made into gruel.

Section 11

Expectorants, Antitussives and Antiasthmatics

This kind of drugs whose principal effects are to remove the stagnation of sputum and alleviate or relieve cough and asthma belongs to the categories of expectorants, antitussives and antiasthmatics of dietetic Chinese drugs.

These drugs are chiefly indicated for cough with abundant sputum, dyspnea due to retention of phlegm, or difficulty in expectoration, and diseases induced by phlegm such as epilepsy, convulsion, goiter, scrofula, deep—rooted carbuncle of yin nature and metastatic abscesses, and cough and asthma due to affection by exopathogenic factors and impairment of the functions of internal organs. They should be chosen in accordance with different syndromes. Other drugs shoud be used together with it according to the cause of disease, too.

For cough due to affection by exopathogens, diaphoretics should be used as well; for cough due to consumptive diseases, tonics should be added; for heat—phlegm syndrome with sticky sputum, it is preferable to use heat-clearing and lung—moistening drugs too; for cold—damp—phlegm syndrome, drugs for drying and warming the lung to expell pathogenic cold—dampness should be added; for cough with hemoptysis, drastic and irritating sputum—resolving drugs should not be used because they might induce or aggravate hemoptysis.

White Mustard seed

ORIGIN The seed of Sinapis alba L., family Cruciferae.

NATURE, TASTE AND CHANNEL TROPISM Acrid in taste, warm

in nature, and attributive to lung channel.

EFFICIENCIES 1. Warm the lung, promote energy circulation and eliminate phlegm.

2. Eliminate phlegm, disperse lumps, dredge the channels and alleviate pain.

INDICATIONS 1. For cold—phlegm and phlegm—retention syndrome with productive cough, thin expectoration, dyspnea, fullness and pain in the chest.

2. For metastatic abscesses due to phlegm—dampness, deep—rooted carbuncle of yin type, numbness and pain of the extremities due to stagnation of phlegm in the channels, and goiter.

DIRECTIONS Decoction: 3—9g.

Bitter Apricot Kernel

ORIGIN Seed of Prunus armeniaca L. var. ansu Maxim. or P. armeniaca L., family Rosaceae.

NATURE, TASTE AND CHANNEL TROPISM Bitter in taste, warm in nature, slightly toxic, and attributive to lung and large intestine channels.

EFFICIENCIES Relieve cough and dyspnea, moisturize the intestine and relax the bowels.

INDICATIONS 1. For wind—heat type, wind—cold type, dryness—heat type cough.

2. For dyspnea due to failure of descending of lung-energy.

3. For constipation due to dryness of intestine.

DIRECTIONS Decoction: 3—9g (crushed before decocting).

Japanese Sea Tangle

ORIGIN The thalline of Laminaria japonica Aresch., family Larminariaceae.

NATURE, TASTE AND CHANNEL TROPISM Bitter and salty in taste, cold in nature, and attributive to liver, stomach and kidney channels.

EFFICIENCIES Eliminate phlegm and soften the hard lumps. Promote diuresis and reduce edema, Lower blood pressure.

INDICATIONS For beriberi, edema, subcutaneous, nodules, scrofula, goiter, tumor and hypertension.

DIRECTIONS Decoction: 9—15g.

CAUTION Contraindicated for spleen—deficiency with loose stools.

Kelp

ORIGIN The whole grass of Zostera marina, family Zosteraceae.

NATURE AND TASTE Salty in taste and cold in nature.

EFFICIENCIES Softening indurated mass and resolving phlegm, inducing diuresis and expelling pathogenic heat.

INDICATIONS It is used to treat goiter, tumor, tuberculosis, mass in the abdomen, hydrops and beriberi. Nowadays it is used mostly to treat simple goiter.

DIRECTIONS To be decocted, boiled, steamed for oral adminitration, or used as an ingredient of a prescription.

Sea Weed

ORIGIN The thalline of Sargassum fusiforme (Harv.) Setch. and S. pallidum (Turn.) C. Ag., family Fueaceae.

NATURE, TASTE AND CHANNEL TROPISE Bitter and salty in taste, cold in nature, and attributive to liver, stomach and kidney channels.

EFFICIENCIES Eliminate phlegm and soften the hard lumps, promote diuresis and reduce edema, lower blood pressure.

INDICATIONS 1. For subcutaneous nodule, scrofula, goiter, tumor, and swelling of testis.

2. For beriberi, edema and hypertension.

DIRECTION Decpoction: 9—15g.

Ginkgo Seed

ORIGIN　The seed (removed off the outer spermoderm) of Ginkgo biloba L., family Ginkgoaceae.

NATURE, FLAVOR AND CHANNEL TROPISM　Sweet, acrid and astringent in taste, mild in nature, slightly toxic, and attributive to lung channel.

EFFICIENCIES　Astringe the lung and relieve dyspnea, clear away turbid substance and decrease frequency of micturition.

INDICATIONS　1. For dyspnea and cough.

2. For leucorrhagia, white and turbid urine, frequent micturition and nocturmal emission.

DIRECTIONS　Decoction: 6—9g.

It should be decocted for a longer time. Crude seed or large dosage may cause poisoning which manifests as vomiting, abdominal pain, diarrhea, coma, somnolence, convulsion, fever, dyspnea, cyanosis, etc., or even death. For moderate toxicosis, decoction of 30g of Ginkgo outer spermoderm or 60g of Radix Glycyrrhizae, or 0.3g of Moschus may be applied.

Lequat Fruit

ORIGIN　Fruit of Eriobotrya japonica (Thunb.) Lindl., family Rosaceae.

NATURE, TASTE AND CHANNEL TROPISM　Bitter in taste, mild in nature, and attributive to lung and stomach channels.

EFFICIENCIES　1. Clear away lung—heat, eliminate phlegm, lower the adverse rising energy and relieve cough.

2. Regulate the stomach to stop vomiting.

INDICATIONS　1. For wind—heat or dryness—heat syndrome manifested as productive cough with thick expectoration, or with dyspnea.

2. For vomiting and thirst due to stomach—heat.

DIRECTION　Decoction: 6—12g.

Peanut

ORIGIN　The seed of Arachis hypogaea, family Leguminosae.

NATURE, FLAVOR AND CHANNEL TROPISM　Sweet in flavor and

neutral in nature,acting on the channels of the spleen and lung.

EFFICIENCIES Moistening the lung,regulating the stomach and arresting bleeding.

INDICATIONS It is used to treat dry cough,regurgitation,beriberi and hypogalactia,and now is used to treat bleeding diseases of the internal organs and hemophilia.

DIRECTIONS To be eaten raw,parched,cooked,or decocted for oral administration. Those who suffer from stagnancy of dampness—cold and lingering diarrhea should not eat it.

The Shoot of Mao Bamboo

ORIGIN The shoot of Phyllostachys pubescens,family Poaceae.

NATURE, TASTE AND CHANNEL TROPISM Sweet in taste and cold in nature,acting on the channels of the large intestine,lung and stomach.

EFFICIENCIES Clearing away heat, resolving phlegm, regulating the function of the stomach and spleen,moisturizing the intestinal tract.

INDICATIONS It is used to treat excessive accumulation of phlegm and heat in the lung,abdominal distention due to retention of food in the stomach, dyschesia,measles reluctant to erupt.

DIRECTIONS To be decocted, eaten cooked or sauted. Children with symptoms of deficiency of the spleen should not eat it excessively.

Section 12

Drugs for Calming the Liver

This kind of drugs whose principal effects are calming the liver to check endogenous wind and relieve convulsion and calming the liver to suppress hyperactivity of the liver—yang belongs to the category of dietetic Chinese drugs for calming the liver.

These drugs are chiefly indicated for dizziness and blurred vision due to hyperactivity of the liver—yang, and spasms and convulsions due to up—stirring of endogenous wind resulting from disorders of the liver. Some drugs in this class also have the effects of clearing away heat from the liver and are therefore effective for blood—shot, swollen and painful eyes and headache due to intense heat in the liver.

Oyster Shell

ORIGIN The shell of Ostrea gigas Thunberg, O. talienwhanensis Crosse or O. rivularis Gould, family Ostreidae.

NATURE, TASTE AND CHANNEL TROPISM Salty and astringent in taste, slightly cold in nature, and attributive to liver and kidney channels.

EFFICIENCIES Calm the liver, benefit yin and suppress the sthenic yang, Soften the hard lumps and disperse the stagnated mass, astringe, invigorate the kidney to preserve essence, antacid and analgesic.

INDICATIONS 1. For sthenia of liver—yang and deficiency of yin leading to hyperactivity of yang manifested as dizziness, tinnitus, irritability and insomnia, convulsion due to affection of wind originated from sthenic liver—yang and febrile diseases with consumption of yin.

2. For subcutaneous nodule, scrofula and goiter.

3. For kidney—deficiency syndrome manifested as emission, enuresis, menorrhagia, metrorrhagia, spontaneous perspiration and night sweat.

4. For peptic ulcer.

INDICATIONS Decoction: 15—30g (crushed and decocted first). Powder: 2—3g tid. External use: Appropriate amount.

Antelope's Horn

ORIGIN The horn of Saiga tatarica L., family Bovidae.

NATURE, TASTE AND CHANNEL TROPISM Salty in taste, cold in nature, and attributive to liver and heart channels.

EFFICIENCIES Clear away heat and calm the liver, expel wind and relieve spasm; Clear away liver—fire to improve visual acuity; Clear away heat and toxic material.

INDICATIONS 1. For heat syndrome with convulsion, hyperactivity or wind transformation of liver—yang with dizziness, numbness and tremor of extremities and convulsion. for severe liver—fire syndrome manifested as epilepsy and insanity.

2. For conjunctivitis and headache.

3. For febrile diseases with coma, delirium and mania.

DIRECTIONS Decoction: 1—3g as slices decocted separately. Juice: 0.5—1.0g prepared by grinding. Powder: 0.5—1.0g.

Celery

ORIGIN The whole grass of Apium graveolens, family Umbelliferae.

NATURE, TASTE AND CHANNEL TROPISM Sweet and bitter in taste and cool in nature, acting on the channels of the stomach and liver.

EFFICIENCIES Calming the liver and clearing away heat, expelling wind and removing dampness by diuresis.

INDICATIONS It is used to treat hypertension, vertigo, headache, flushed face, conjunctival congestion, dysentery with bloody stool, carbuncle and swelling.

DIRECTIONS To be eaten sauteed, or decocted for oral administration; or to be pounded to get its juice or mashed for external application.

Section 13

Tranquilizers

This kind of drugs whose principal effects are tranquilizing the mind and relieving uneasiness belongs to the category of tranquilizers of dietetic Chinese drugs.

Tranquilizers exert tranquilizing effects either through sedation or through noruishment of the heart. They are chiefly used in the treatment of irritability, palpitation or svere palpitation, insomnia and dreaminess due to deficiency of the heart—qi and insufficiency of the heart—blood, or due to exuberant fire resulting from hyperactivity of the heart. They are also used to treat such diseases as infantile convulsion, epilepsy and mania.

Drugs of this class can be selected for use according to the etiology and pathogenesis of the disease and used together with suitable drugs of other classes. For syndrome due to deficiency of yin and insufficiency of the blood, drugs for nourishing the blood and strengthening yin should be added; for syndrome due to exuberant fire caused by hyperactivity of the heart, drugs for removing excessive fire from the heart should be given as well.

Wild Jujube Seed

ORIGIN Seed of Ziziphus spinosa Hu, family Rhamnaceae.

NATURE, TASTE AND CHANNEL TROPLSM Sweet and sour in taste, mild in nature, and attributive to heart and liver channels.

EFFICIENCIES Nourish the heart, benefit the liver and tranquilize the mind and stop sweating.

INDICATIONS 1. For deficiency of heart—blood and liver—blood with vexation, insomnia, severe palpitation, frightening and amnesia, liver—deficiency with heat, yin—deficiency with yang—hyperactivity.

2. For general debility with spontaneous perspiration, and night sweating.

DIRECTIONS Decoction: 9—18g.

Section 14

Digestives

The kind of drugs whose principal action is to improve appetite and digestion and remove food stagnation, is referred to as digestives of dietetic Chinese drugs.

Drugs of this class can remove stagnated food and restore normal functions of the spleen and stomach in transporting and distributing nutrients. They are indicated for abdominal distension, belching, acid regurgitation, nausea, vomiting, and irregular bowel movements due to indigestion and food retention. They are also effective for indigestion due to the weakness of the spleen and stomach.

Hawthorn Fruit

ORIGIN　Fruit of Crataegus pinnatifida Bunge, and C. cuneata Sieb. et Zucc., family Rosaceae.

NATURE, TASTE AND CHANNEL TROPISM　Both are sour and sweet in taste, slightly warm in nature, and attributive to spleen, stomach and liver channels.

EFFICIENCIES　1. Strengthen the stomach and improve digestion, relieve diarrhea and dysentery, promote blood circulation and disperse blood stasis, lower blood pressure and the level of blood lipids.

INDICATIONS　1. For dyspepsia, especially over feeding in infants and immoderate eating of meats.

2. For diarrhea and dysentery, expecially for those caused by immoderate eating and drinking.

3. For blood—stasis syndrome manifested as anemia, postpartum abdominal pain with lochiostasis, angina pectoris, polyp of vocal cord; also for inguinal hernia or swelling of testis with bearing—down pain, hepatosplenomegaly, and cystic hyperplasia of the breast.

4. For hypertension and hyperlipidemia.

DIRECTIONS　Decoction: 6—12g; 30—60g for anemia, angina pectoris, polyp of vocal cord, hypertension and hyperlipidemia: also as gargle for polyp of vocal cord.

Germinated

ORIGIN The germinant fruit of Hordeum vulgare L. ,family Gramineae.

NATURE,TASTE AND CHANNEL TROPISM Sweet in taste,warm in nature,and attributive to spleen and stomach channels.

EFFICIENCIES Strengthen the stomach and improve digestion and be lactifuge.

INDICATIONS 1. For dyspepsia of starches,vomiting of milk in infants caused by improper feeding,and anorexia due to deficiency of spleen and stomach.

2. For galactostasis and as lactifuge for breast—feeding women.

DIRECTIONS Decoction: 10—15g; 60—120g of fresh sample for lactifuge.

Rice Sprout

ORIGIN Fruit of Oryza sativa L. ,family Gramineae.

NATURE,TASTE AND CHANNEL TROPISM Sweet in taste,warm in nature,and attributive to spleen and stomach channels.

EFFICIENCIES Strengthen the stomach and promote digestion.

INDICATIONS For dyspepsia of starches and anorexia with deficiency of spleen and stomach.

DIRECTION Decoction:10—15g.

Membrane of Chicken's Gizzard

ORIGIN The membrane of the gizzard of Gallus gallus domesticus Brisson,family phasianidae.

NATURE,TASTE AND CHANNEL TROPISM Sweet intaste,mild in nature,and attributive to stomach,spleen,small in testine and urinary bladder channels.

EFFICIENCIES Strengthen the stomach and improve digestion,relieve nocturnal emission,disperse blood stasis and eliminate stones.

INDICATIONS 1. Single use for dyspepsia with vomiting or infantile vomiting after immoderate feeding; for indigestion with spleen—deficiency; for infantile malnutrition involving the spleen.

2. For emission and enuresis due to kidney—deficiency.

3. For hepatosplenomegaly, dyspepsia and anemia, for urinary and biliary stones.

DIRECTIONS Decoction: 3—9g Powder: 1—3g tid for dyspepsia.

Radish Seed

ORIGIN Seed of Raphanus sativus L., family Cruciferae.

NATURE, TASTE AND CHANNEL TROPISM Acrid and sweet in taste, mild in nature, and attributive to lung, spleen and stomach channels.

EFFICIENCIES Promote digestion and relieve dyspepsia. eliminate phlegm and descend the adverse—rising energy, lower blood pressure.

INDICATIONS 1. For serious cases of dyspepsia with chest upset, abdominal distension, eructation, acid regurgitation, constipation, or diarrhea.

2. For productive cough, dyspnea and hypertension.

DIRECTIONS Decoction: 6—12g, 15—30g for constipation of sthenia-syndrome; 50—70g for hypertension.

Powder: 9—12g for habitual constipation.

Carrot

ORIGIN The root of Daucus carota, family Umbelliferae.

NATURE, TASTE AND CHANNEL TROPISM Sweet in taste, neutral in nature, and attributive to lung and spleen channels.

EFFICIENCIES Strengthening the spleen and removing stagnation of food.

INDICATIONS It is used for treatment of maldigestion, protracted dysentery and cough.

DIRRECTIONS To be eaten either raw or cooked. It will strenghten and tonify the five viscera, promote digestion, nourish the kidney—yin, and invigorate the kidney—yang to eat carrot for a long period of time.

Radish

ORIGIN The fresh root of Raphanus sativus, family Cruciferae.

NATURE, TASTE AND CHANNEL TROPISM Pungent, sweet in taste, cool in nature, and attributive to lung and stomach channels.

EFFICIENCIES Removing food stagnation, clearing away phlegm—heat, keeping the adverse qi flowing downward, regulating the middle—jiao, clearing away toxic materials.

INDICATIONS It is used to treat food stagnation, turgor, aphonia caused by cough due to accumulation of phlegm, hematemesis, nose—bleeding, diabetes, dysentery, megrim and headache.

DIRECTIONS To be eaten raw, stir—fried, cooked, or made into medicated diet. It can also be decocted or pounded to get its juice for drinking, or applied to the affected part when used externally. Patients manifesting symptoms of insufficiency of the spleen—yang should not eat it.

Section 15

Anthelmintics

This kind of drugs which can expel or poison parasites is referred to as anthelmintics of dietetic Chinese drugs.

Anthelmintics are indicated for diseases caused by parasites in the intestines, such as ascariasis, enterobiasis, cestodiasis and ancylostomiasis.

Anthelmintics should be selected for specific parasites and supplemented with other types of suitable drugs according to the actual condition.

Chinese Torreya

ORIGIN Seed of Torreya grandis Fort., family Taxaceae.

NATURE, TASTE AND CHANNEL TROPISM Sweet in taste, mild in nature, and attributive to stomach and large intestine channels.

EFFICIENCIES Kill parasite and laxative.

INDICATIONS For ascariasis and taeniasis, also for constipation due to dryness of intestine.

DIRECTIONS For parasitic infestation: 15—30g (fried) for chewing, or prepared as pill or powder.

For constipation: Fresh sample prepared as powder.

Pumpkin Seed

ORIGIN Seed of Cucurbita moschata Duch., family Cucurbitaceae.

NATURE, TASTE AND CHANNEL TROPISM Sweet in taste, warm in nature, and attributive to stomach and large intestine channels.

EFFICIENCIES Kill parasite.

INDICATIONS 1. For taeniasis.

2. For schistosomiasis, symptomatic relief (including the fever subsidence in acute infection) is evident, but the ova negative rate is not high; also for ascariasis.

DIRECTIONS For taeniasis: 60—120g as powder.

For schistosomiasis: 200—300g daily, prepare as aqueous extract or as decoction with oily component discarded, for one month.

For ascariasis: 30—60g chewed and swallowed for 1—3 days in children.

Section 16

Tonics

This kind of drugs which can tonify the deficient qi, blood, yin and yang of the body, enhance the body resistance to diseases, and be used in the treatment of various deficiency syndromes are known as tonics of dietetic Chinese drugs.

These drugs in accordance with their action are divided into four types: drugs for tonifying qi, yang, blood and yin. Drugs for tonifying qi of this type can invigorate the physiological function of the body, and are mainly indicated for qi deficiency syndromes, especially effective for deficiency of the spleen—qi characterized by anorexia, loose stool, gastric and abdominal distension, lack of vitality, lassitude, edema, prolapse of rectum, and deficiency of the lung—qi characterized by short breath, disinclination to talk, breathlessness after movement, spontaneous sweating, etc.

Yang tonics of this type are mainly indicated for yang deficiency syndromes which include deficiency of the heart—yang, deficiency of the spleen—yang and deficiency of the kidney—yang, and function in reinforcing the kidney—yang, tonifying the essence of life and strengthening the bones and muscles. They are usually used for syndrome of deficiency of the kidney—yang manifested as aversion to cold, cold limbs, aches and lassitude or cold pain in the loins and knees, impotence, spermatorrhea, sterility due to uterine coldness, lucid and thin leucorrhagia, frequent urination, enuresis, deep pulse, white tongue coating, etc.

Blood tonic of this type have the effects of tonifying the blood and are indicated for syndromes of blood deficiency shown as sallow complexion, paleness of the lips, tongue and nails, dizziness, blurred vision, palpitation, delayed menstrual cycle with scanty pale menstrual blood, or even amenorrhea, etc.

Yin tonic of this type function in tonifying the yin fluid, and promoting the production of body fluid to moisten dryness. They are indicated for deficiency of the lung—yin manifested as dry cough with little sputum and dryness of the mouth and tongue; deficiency of the stomach—yin manifested as red tongue with little coating, dry throat and thirsty feeling; deficiency of the liver—yin characterized by blurred vision and xenophthalmia of the eyes, dizziness and tinnitus; and deficiency of the kidney—yin with manifestations of lassitude of the loins and legs, seminal emission, night sweat, etc.

Because the qi, blood, yin and yang in the human body are interdependent, deficiency of yang is often accompanied with deficiency of qi, and in turn, deficiency of qi is most likely to develop into or lead to deficiency of yang. The deficiency of yang and qi indicates the physiological hypofunction of the body. Similarly, deficiency of yin is usually accompanied with deficiency of blood and deficiency of blood is liable to cause deficiency of yin. Deficiency of blood and yin indicates the consumption of vital essence, blood and body fluid. For these reasons, drugs for tonifying qi and yang and drugs for tonifying blood and yin are often used together for mutual reinforcement. In case deficiency of qi and blood occurs, or deficiency of yin and yang exists at the same time, a therapy of tonifying both qi and blood, or both yin and yang, should be recommended.

Because they are effective for deficiency, tonics should not be abused. Otherwise they may give rise to other problems. In case that pathogens of excess type are still present and there is no sign of deficiency of the vital qi, tonics should not be used so as to avoid any interference in the elimination of pathogens which may aggravate the condition, therefore, they are used over a long period of time, some of the tonics may impede digestion, so they can be supplemented with drugs for strengthening the spleen and stomach, and qi tonic are tending to give rise to accumulation of qi shown as distension and fullness in the chest and abdomen and anorexia, qi tonics should be used with small amounts of drugs for promoting circulation of qi and digestion.

Most of the yang tonics are warm and dry in property and can hurt yin and increase pathogenic fire, so they should not be used in case of hyperactivity of fire due to deficiency of yin.

Pilose Antler

ORIGIN　The horn of the male beast of Cervus nippon, family Cerridae.

NATURE, TASTE AND CHANNEL TROPISM　Sweet and salty in taste, warm in nature, and attributive to kidney and liver channels.

EFFICIENCIES　Invigorate kidney—yang, supplement essence and blood and strengthen the tendons and bones.

INDICATIONS　For deficiency of kidney—yang manifested as cold limbs, fatigue, backache, impotence, emission and frequent micturition, enuresis, sterility, metrorrhagia or leucorrhagia; for hypofunction of kidney with shortness of breath and dyspnea; for yang—deficiency and insufficiency of essence and blood manifested as flaccidity of extremities, or maldevelopment, delayed walking, delayed teeth eruption and delayed closure of fontanel in infants, or unhealed skin lesions.

DIRECTIONS Pill or powder: 0. 25—0. 5g bid or tid.

Fresh—Water Turtle Shell

ORIGIN The shell of Trionyx sinensis Wiegmann, family Trionychidae.

NATURE, TASTE AND CNALLEN TROPISM Salty in taste, slightly cold in nature, and attributive to liver and kidney channels.

EFFICIENCIES Nourish yin and suppress the sthenic yang, soften and disperse the lumps.

INDICATIONS For yin—deficiency with hyperactivity of asthenic fire manifested as hectic fever and night sweating; or for the late stage of febrile diseases with consumption of yin fluid manifested as night fever; or for convulsion of yin—deficiency type.

2. For abdominal mass; recently, used for hepatosplenomegaly.

DIRECTIONS Decoction: 10—30g (decocted first).

Donkey—hide

ORIGIN Donkey hide stewed and concentrated as gelatinous masses, of Equus asinus, family Equidae.

NATURE, TASTE AND CHANNEL TROPISM Sweet in taste, mild in nature, and attributive to lung, liver and kidney channels.

EFFICIENCIES Enrich blood and stop bleeding, regulate the menstruation and soothe the fetus, and nouish yin and moisturize the lung.

INDICATIONS 1. For blood—deficiency with sallow complexion, dizzsiness and palpitation; for asthenia—syndrome manifested as various types of bleeding, such as hemoptysis, hematemesis, hemafecia, hematuria, metrorrhagia, etc. Recently, used for anemia, leukocytopenia and thrombocytopenic purpura.

2. For blood—deficiency syndrome manifested as menoxenia, anemia, and threatened abortion.

3. For febrile diseases with consumption of yin or yin—deficiency with fire—hyperactivity manifested as vexation and insomnia; insufficiency of yin—blood with muscular spasm; dryness of the lung with cough and thirst.

DIRECTION Dissolved 6—9g with the decoction.

Walnut Kernel

ORIGIN Seed of Juglans regia L. ,family Juglandaceae.

NATURE, TASTE AND CHANNEL TROPISM Sweet in taste, warm in nature, and attributive to lung, kidney and large intestine channels.

EFFICIENCIES Invigorate kidney—yang and strengthen the waist and knees, invigorate the lung and relieve dyspnea, moisturize the intestine and relax bowels.

INDICATIONS 1. For deficiency of kidney—yang with soreness and weakness of the waist and knees, frequent micturition and enuresis.

2. For lung—deficiency or deficiency of the lung and kidney with dyspneic cough.

3. For constipation due to dryness of the intestine and consumption of body fluid. In addition, also used for urinary calculus. Its paste or oil preparations be applied topically for dermatitis and eczema.

DIRECTIONS Decoction: 10—30g; 30—100g fried with sesame oil and taken with 30g of sugar in two to three divided doses daily.

Placenta Hominis

ORIGIN The normal placenta of Homo Sapiens L. , family Hominidae. Prepared by removing the amnion, umbilical cord and blood, and drying after cooked.

NATURE, TASTE AND CHANNEL TROPISM Sweet and salty in taste, warm in nature, and attributive to heart, lung and kidney channels.

EFFICIENCIES Invigorate the kidney and supplement essence, invigorate vital energy and enrich blood, and invigorate the lung and relieve cough.

INDICATIONS 1. For insufficiency of kidney—yang and kidney—essence manifested as sterility, impotence, emission, dizziness and tinnitus.

2. For insufficiency of vital energy and blood manifested as shortness of breath, fatigue, poor appetite, and galactoschesis; for the debilitated who are sus-

ceptable to common cold and skin infection.

3. For lung—deficiency or deficiency of the lung, spleen and kidney with dyspneic cough.

DIRECTION Pill or powder: 1.5—2.0g bid or tid.

Bitter Cardamon

ORIGIN Fruit of Alpinia oxyphylla Miq., family Zingiberaceae.

NATURE, TASTE AND CHANNEL TROPISM Acrid in taste, warm in nature, and attributive to spleen and kidney channels.

EFFICIENCIES Warm the spleen and preserve saliva, preserve essence and decrease micturition.

INDICATIONS 1. For spleen deficiency with salivation.

2. For cold—dampness of spleen and kidney manifested as abdominal pain, vomiting and diarrhea.

3. For deficiency—cold of kidney energy manifested as nocturnal emission, enuresis, nocturia, or slow and difficult discharge of urine.

DIRECTION Decoction: 3—6g.

Lily Bulb

ORIGIN The scale leaf of the bulb of Lilium lancifolium Thunb. or several species of the same genus, family Liliaceae.

NATURE, TASTE AND CHANNEL TROPISM Slightly bitter in taste, mild in nature, and attributive to heart and lung channels.

EFFICIENCIES Moisturize the lung and relieve cough, clear away heart—fire and tranquilize the mind.

INDICATIONS 1. For lung—dryness with cough and hemoptysis.

2. For the convalescence of febrile diseases or yin—deficiency with heat manifested as irritability, insomnia, dreaminess, palpitation and absent—mindedness.

DIRECTIONS Decoction: 10—30g.

Wolfberry Fruit

ORIGIN Fruit of Lycium barbarum L. ,family Solanaceae.

NATURE,TASTE AND CHANNEL TROPISM Sweet in taste,mild in nature,and attributive to liver and kidney channels.

EFFICIENCIES Nourish yin,enrich blood,benefit essence and improve visual acuity.

INDICATIONS For deficiency of liver—yin and kidney—yin and insufficiency of essence and blood manifested as dizziness,blurring of vision,hypopsia, tinnitus,emission and soreness of the loin and extremities,also for diabetes.

DIRECTIONS Decoction:6—15g.

Longan Aril

ORIGIN The aril of Euphoria longan (Lour.) Steud. , family Sapindaceae.

NATURE,TASTE AND CHANNEL TROPISM Sweet in taste,warm in nature,and attributive to heart and spleen channels.

EFFICIENCIES Invigorate the heart and spleen,nourish blood and calm the mind.

INDICATIONS For deficiency of vital energy and blood manifested as palpitation,insomnia,amnesia and dizziness,or during convalescence and after delivery.

DIRECTION Decoction:6—15g;up to 30—60g.

Tortoise Plastron

ORIGIN The plastron of Chinemys reevesii(Gray),family Testudinidae.

NATURE, TASTE AND CHANNEL TROPISM Sour and sweet in taste,slightly cold in nature,and attributive to kidney and liver channels.

EFFICIENCIES Nourish yin and suppress the sthenic yang. benefit kidney and invigorate bone,regulate menstruation and relieve metrorrhagia.

INDICATIONS 1. For yin—deficiency with fire hyperactivity manifested as hectic fever, night sweat, nocturnal emission, dizziness and tinnitus, yin—deficiency with wind hyperactivity manifested as convulsion.

2. For hypofunction of liver and kidney manifested as flaccidity of the waist and lower limbs, weakness of the tendons and bones, delayed ability of standing and walking, delayed growth of teeth and delayed closure of fontanel in infants.

3. For yin—deficiency with blood—heat manifested as metrorrhagia, menorrhagia and leucorrhagia.

DIRECTION Decoction: 10—30g (decocted first).

Liquorice

ORIGIN Root of Glycyrrhiza uralensis Fisch. or G. glabra L., family Leguminosae.

NATURE, TASTE AND CHANNEL TROPISM Sweet in taste, mild in nature, and attributive to spleen and stomach channels.

EFFICIENCIES Invigorate vital energy, clear away heat and toxic material, eliminate phlegm and relieve cough, relieve spasm and alleviate pain, and moderate the potency of drugs.

INDICATIONS 1. For syndrome of spleen—stomach dificiency; for those with deficiency of vital energy, for those with yang—deficiency for those with deficiency of heart energy or heart—yang manifested as shortness of breath, palpitation, chest pain and irrhythmia.

2. For serious heat—syndrome such as skin infection, sore throat, etc. or drug and food poisoning.

3. For various types of cough and dyspnea.

4. For spasm and pain of the abdomen and leg, arthralgia of wind—dampness—cold type and peptic ulcer.

5. For counteracting the toxicity or side effects of potent drugs such as Radix et Rhizoma Rhei, Radix Aconiti Praeparata, Radix Aconiti, etc. Also used for adjusting the taste of drugs. Recently, used for virus hepatitis, thrombocytopenic purpura and anaphylactoid purpura.

DIRECTIONS Decoction: 3—9g; up to 30g for heart—energy deficiency, food and drug poisoning.

CAUTION 1. Edema and hypertension may ensue after a long period of administration.

2. Incompatible with Radix Euphorbiae Kansui, Flos Genkwa, and Radix Euphorbice Pekinensis, etc.

Mulberry

ORIGIN Fruit of Morus alba L., family Moraceae.

NATURE, TASTE AND CHANNEL TROPISM Sweet and sour in taste, warm in nature, and attributive to heart, liver and kidney channels.

EFFICIENCIES Nourish yin, enrich blood, moisturize dryness and calm the wind.

INDICATIONS For insufficiency of yin—blood or stirring up of wind—yang manifested as dizziness, tinnitus, vexation and insomnia; for diabetes due to yin—deficiency and insufficiency of fluid; for constipation due to deficiency of yin and dryness of intestine. Recently, used for anemia, neurasthenia, diabetes mellitus and hypertension of yin—deficiency type.

DIRECTIONS Decoction: 15—30g.

Chinese Date

ORIGIN Fruit of Ziziphus jujuba Mill., family Rhamnmaceae.

NATURE, TASTE AND CHANNEL TROPISM Sweet in taste, warm in nature, and attributive to spleen and stomach channels.

EFFICIENCIES Invigorate the spleen and stomach, nourish blood and calm the mind, moderate the potency of drugs.

INDICATIONS 1. For deficiency of spleen and stomach with poor appetite, fatigue and loose stools.

2. For blood—deficiency with insomnia, vexation and restlessness.

3. For counteracting the toxicity of side effects of potent drugs, such as Flos Genkwa, Radix Euphorbiae Pekinensis, Semen Lepidii seu Descurainiae, etc. Recently, also used for anaphylactoid purpura and bronchial asthma.

DIRECTION Decoction:10—30g.

Dogwood Fruit

ORIGIN The pulp of Cornus officinalis Sieb. et Zucc. ,family Comaceae.

NATURE,TASTR AND CHANNEL TROPISM Sour and astringent in taste,slightly warm in nature,and attributive to liver and kidney channels.

EFFICIENCIES Invigorate the liver and kidney,supplement the essence and improve visual acuity,astringe and preserve essence.

INDICATIONS 1. For deficiency of the liver and kidney manifested as soreness of the waist and knees,flaccidity of lower limbs,impotence,frequent micturition,sterility,dizziness,tinnitus and blurring of vision.

2. For hypofunction of liver and kindey manifested as emission,enuresis,frequent micturition,metrorrhagia,menorrhagia,spontaneous perspiration,night sweat,collapse with profuse perspiration and dyspnea of asthenic type.

DIRECTION Decoction:6—12g,up to 30g.

Hyacinth Bean

ORIGIN Seed of Dolichos lablab L. ,family Leguminosae.

NATURE,TASTE CNANNEL TROPISM Sweet and bland in taste, mild in nature,and attributive to spleen and stomach channels.

EFFICIENCIES Invigorate the spleen and deprive dampness.

INDICATIONS For deficiency of spleen and stomach manifested as poor appetite,loose stools or diarrhea,leucorrhagia,fried sample is more suitable;for affection of summer—heat and dampness manifested as vomiting,diarrhea,feeling of oppression in the chest,fresh sample is more suitable.

DIRECTION Decoction:9—18g.

Chinese Yam

ORIGIN Rhizome of Dioscorea opposita Thunb. ,family Dioscoreaceae.

NATURE, TASTE AND CHANNEL TROPISM Sweet in taste, mild in nature, and attributive to spleen, lung and kidney channels.

EFFICIENCIES Invigorate the spleen and stomach, invigorate the lung, and invigorate the kidney and preserve the essence.

INDICATIONS 1. For deficiency of spleen-energy and stomach—energy with poor appetite, fatigue, loose stools or chronic diarrhea, leucorrhagia, etc. ; for febrile diseases with consumption of body fluid or deficiency of spleen—yin and stomach—yin with poor appetite, thirst, dry tongue, diabetes, etc.

2. For lung—deficiency with chronic cough or tuberculosis; for deficiency of lung and kidney with dyspnea and chronic cough.

3. For kidney—deficiency manifested as emission, enuresis, frequent micturition and leucorrhagia.

DIRECTION Decoction: 10-30g

Crystal Sugar

ORIGIN The ice—like rock crystal boiled and crystallized out of white granulated sugar.

NATURE, TASTR AND CHANNEL TROPISM Sweet in flavor, neutral in nature, acting on the channels of the lung and spleen.

EFFICIENCIES Invigorating the middle—jiao and replenishing qi, regulating the function of the stomach and moistening the lung.

INDICATIONS It is used to treat cough and asthma due to dryness of the lung, deficiency of the lung, wind—cold pathogen and overwork; infantile malaria, fasting dysentery, aphthae; toothache due to pathogenic windfire.

DIRECTIONS To be decocted for internal use, or eaten together with rice or bread. It can be used as an ingredient of boluses or pills or soft extract.

Pear

ORIGIN Mainly the cultivar fruit of Pyrus brets—chneideri, P. pyrifolia and P. ussuriensis, family Rosaceae.

NATURE, TASTE AND CHANNEL TROPISM Sweet, slightly sour in

flavor and cool in nature,acting on the channels of the lung and stomach.

EFFICIENCIES Promoting the production of body fluid,moistening dryness,clearing away pathogenic heat and resolving phlegm.

INDICATIONS It is used to treat restlessness and thirst due to impairment of the body fluid during febrile diseases, xiaoke (including diabetes), cough of heat type, madness by fright due to phlegm — heat, dysphagia and constipation.

DIRECTIONS To be eaten raw, pounded (after peeled and stoned) to get its juice, boiled down to jelly, or decocted for oral administration. Those who suffer from loose stools caused by insufficiency of the spleen should avoid it.

Milk

ORIGIN The milk of Bos taurus domesticus of Bubalus bubalis, family Bovidae.

NATURE, TASTE AND CHANNEL TROPISM Sweet in taste and neutral in nature, acting on the channels of the heart, lung and stomach.

EFFICIENCIES Treating consumptive disease, reinforcing the lung and stomach, promoting the production of body fluid and moistening the intestinal tract.

INDICATIONS It is used to treat debility and internal injury caused by overstrain, regurgitation, dysphagia, diabetes and constipation.

DIRECTIONS To be taken after boiling or sterilization. Precaution should be taken by patients suffering from diarrhea caused by insufficiency of the spleen —yang or fluid—retention or phlegm—dampness in the body.

Cushaw

ORIGIN The fruit of Cucurbita moschata, family Cucurbitaceae.

NATURE, TASTE AND CHANNEL TROPISM Sweet in taste and warm in nature, acting on the channels of the spleen and stomach.

EFFICIENCIES AND INDICATIONS Invigorating the spleen and stomach and replenishing qi, relieving inflammation and pains, removing toxic materials of any substance and destroying intestinal parasites.

DIRECTIONS To be eaten steamed, cooked, or to be decocted for oral administration, or to be mashed for external use. Cushaw has the effects of invigoration, replenishment, alleviation of water retention and inducing diuresis when eaten cooked, but it can expel intestinal ascarides and clear away toxic materials when eaten raw.

Sea Cucumber

ORIGIN The whole of Stichopus japonicus, family Stichopodidae, or any of the other sea cucumbers.

NATURE, TASTE AND CHANNEL TROPISM Salty in taste and warm in nature, acting on the channels of the heart and kidney.

EFFICIENCIES Tonifying the kidney, replenishing the vital essence, nourishing the blood and moistening dryness.

INDICATIONS It is used to treat deficiency of the essence and blood, weakness, impotence and seminal emission, frequent urination, constipation due to dryness of the intestinal tract, and debility of the aged.

DIRECTIONS To be made into soup or eaten sauteed after soaked. Patients suffering from diarrhea due to deficiency of the spleen or excessive phlegm should avoid it.

Eel

ORIGIN The flesh or the whole of Monopterus albus, family Symbranchidae.

NATURE, TASTE AND CHANNEL TROPISM Sweet in taste and warm in nature, acting on the channels of the liver, spleen and kidney.

EFFICIENCIES Treating deficiency syndromes, expelling pathogenic wind and dampness, strengthening the muscles and bones.

INDICATIONS It is used to treat impairment due to consumptive diseases, arthralgia caused by pathogenic wind—cold—dampness, postpartum stranguria, dysentery with pus and blood in the stools, piles and ecthyma.

DIRECTIONS To be boiled in clear soup or steamed, or made into medicated diet. Its flesh can be made into small balls and quick—boiled in boiling clear water. When used externally, it is to be pounded for application to, or sliced to stick on, the affected part.

Chestnut

ORIGIN The shelled seed of Castanea mollissima, family Fagaceae.

NATURE, TASTE AND CHANNEL TROPISM Sweet in taste and warm in nature, acting on the channels of the spleen, stomach and kidney.

EFFICIENCIES Nourishing the stomach and strengthening the spleen, tonifying the kidney to strengthen the muscles, promoting blood circulation and arresting bleeding.

INDICATIONS It is used to treat regurgitation of food from stomach or diarrhea due to weakness of the spleen and stomach, soreness of the waist and weakness of the legs caused by general deficiency of the human body, hematemesis, nose — bleeding, hemafecia, incised wound, ecchymoma and pain resulting from fracture, scrofula and pyogenic infections.

DIRECTIONS To be eaten raw, cooked, parched, or stewed along with meat. It is effective for arresting bleeding to eat it raw; while for invigoration and replenishment, to eat it cooked. Nevertheless excessive eating is no good.

Polished Round Grained Rice

ORIGIN The seed of Oryza sativa, family Gramineae.

NATURE, TASTE AND CHANNEL TROPISM Sweet in taste, warm in nature, and attributive to spleen and stomach channels.

EFFICIENCIES AND INDICATIONS Invigorating the middle—jiao and replenishing qi, strengthening the spleen and regulating the stomach, relieving thirst and restlessness, and arresting dysentery and diarrhea.

DIRECTIONS To be eaten steamed, made into gruels, or compounded into medicated diet or medicated gruel. The patient with endogenous cold should eat less.

Millet

ORIGIN The seed of Setaria italica, family Gramineae.

NATURE, TASTE AND CHANNEL TROPISM Sweet, salty in taste, cool in nature. Old millet is bitter in taste, cold in nature, and attributive to kidney, spleen and stomach channels.

EFFICIENCIES Regulating the middle — jiao, tonifying the kidney, removing pathogenic heat and poisonous quality of any substance.

INDICATIONS It is used to treat fever of deficiency type in the spleen and stomach, regurgitation of food from the stomach and vomiting, diabetes and diarrhea. Old millet can arrest dysentery, relieve thirst and restlessness. Millet is appropriate for treating dripping urination resulting from damp — heat of the spleen, stomach and kidney.

DIRECTIONS To be decocted of made into gruel. Less should be taken by those who are in a morbid condition resulting from insufficiency of genuine qi with endogenous cold manifested as light — coloured urine. Don't rub the seeds with your hands while washing them; avoid either soaking them in water for long or washing them in hot water.

Wheat

ORIGIN The seed or flour of Triticum aestivum, family Gramineae.

NATURE, TASTE AND CHANNEL TROPISM Sweet in taste, cool in nature, and attributive to heart, spleen and kidney channels.

EFFICIENCIES Nourishing the heart, tonifying the kidney, removing pathogenic heat and relieving thirst.

INDICATIONS It is used to treat hysteria, dysphoria, diabetes, diarrhea, dysentery, carbuncle and swelling, bleeding due to injury, and scald.

DIRECTIONS To be decocted, made into gruel or made into cooked wheaten food for oral regular administration; when used externally, it is to be roasted and ground into powder to treat carbuncle and swelling, injuries and scald. Noodles should be avoided by those who are ill with damp — heat syndrome.

SUPPLEMENT Light Wheat: It can arrest sweating and is used to treat excessive sweating due to debility.

Black Sesame

ORIGIN The black seed of Sesamum indicum, family Pedaliaceae.

NATURE, TASTE AND CHANNEL TROPISM Sweet in taste, neutral in nature, and attributive to liver and kidney channels.

EFFICIENCIES Invigorating the liver and kidney, moisturizing the five viscera.

INDICATIONS It is used as a cure of deficiency of both the liver and the kidney, dizziness due to endopathic wind of deficiency type, migratory arthralgia, paralyses, dry stools and difficult defection, weakness during the convalescence, early greying of air, lack of lactation in women.

DIRECTIONS To be decocted, or made into gruel along with polished round—grained rice, or used as an ingredient of boluses, powder for internal use. It can also be decocted for bathing or pounded for external application. It should be avoided by those who suffer from loose stools due to insufficiency of the spleen.

Pork

ORIGIN The meat of Sus scrofa demestica, family Suidae.

NATURE, TASTE AND CHANNEL TROPISM Sweet, salty in taste, neutral in nature, and attributive to spleen, stomach and kidney channels.

EFFICIENCIES Tonifying the kidney, nourishing the blood, replenishing yin—essence and moistening dryness of the viscera.

INDICATIONS It is used for treatment of consumption of yin during the course of febrile diseases, diabetes, emaciation, debility due to deficiency of the kidney, postpartum deficiency of blood, dry cough and constipation.

DIRECTIONS To be eaten sauted, boiled, roasted, or to be made into medicated diet for eating, or made into soup for drinking. Precaution should be taken by patients with symptoms of phlegm and damp—heat accumulated in the body.

SUPPLEMENT Pork Liver: It can tonify the liver, nourish the blood and improve eyesight.

Pork Tripe, i. e. pork stomach: It can tonify consumption, strengthen the spleen and stomach.

Pork Kidney, commonly known as "Zhuyaozi" in Chinese. It is used to treat lumbago resulting from kidney deficiency, hydrops, seminal emission, night sweat and deafness of the aged.

Pork Brain: It is used to treat wind syndrome of head ache, dizziness, frost-bite and rhagas.

Pig Trotters: They can tonify the blood, promote lactation and pus discharge. They are used to treat lack of lactation, boils and suppurative skin diseases.

Mutton

ORIGIN The meat of Capra hircus and Oris aries, family Bovidae.

NATURE, TASTE AND CHANNEL TROPISM Sweet in taste, warm in nature, and attributive to spleen and kidney channels.

EFFICIENCIES Invigorating qi to treat deficiency syndrome, warming the middle—jiao and relaxing the bowels.

INDICATIONS It is used for treatment of magersucht due to consumption, lassitude in the loins and knees, insufficiency—cold syndrome after delivery, abdominal pain, periumbilical colic due to invasion of cold, regurgitation of food from the stomach due to deficiency of the middle—jiao.

DIRECTIONS To be decocted, boiled, sauted for eating. It should be avoided by those who have symptoms caused by exopathy or retained heat in the body.

SUPPLEMENT Goat or Sheep Kidney, also known as "Yang yaozi" in Chinese. It can tonify the kidney—qi, replenish the vital essence and marrow, and is used to treat seminal emission due to deficiency of the kidney, soreness and pain along the spinal column, deafness and tinnitus.

The Milk: Having the effects of warming, moistening and tonifying the human body, it is used for treatment of magersucht due to consumption, diabetes, regurgitation of food from the stomach.

The Liver: It can replenish the blood, tonify the liver and improve eyesight, and is used for treatment of sallow complexion and magersucht due to deficiency of blood, dim eyesight due to deficiency of liver, night blindness, cataract and nebula.

Dog Meat

ORIGIN The meat of Canis familiaris, family Ganidae.

NATURE, TASTE AND CHANNEL TROPISM Salty in taste, warm in nature, and attributive to spleen, stomach and kidney channels.

EFFICIENCIES Reinforcing the functing of the spleen and stomach to benefit qi, warming the kidney to reinforce yang.

INDICATIONS It is used to treat deficiency of qi of the spleen and stomach, fullness sensation and depressed feeling in the chest and abdomen, general edema, lassitude in the loins and knees, long—unhealed obstinate soreness.

DIRECTIONS To be eaten stewed, or decocted for drinking. It is warm—natured, so precaution should be taken by patients with symptoms of interior heat.

SUPPLEMENT Dog Testis, Dog Penis: Being able to tonify the human body and strengthen the kidney, both of them are used to treat impotence due to deficiency of the kidney and postpartum impairment of the kidney due to overstrain that is so severe as if the patient suffered from malaria.

Black—Bone Chicken

ORIGIN The whole substance, except the internal organs, of Gallus domesticus, a kind of chicken.

NATURE, TASTE AND CHANNEL TROPISM Sweet in taste, neutral in nature, and attributive to liver and kidney channels.

EFFICIENCIES　Tonifying the liver and kidney, nourishing yin and bringing down fever.

INDICATIONS　It is used for treatment of hectic fever and magersucht due to consumptive diseases, diabetes, lingering diarrhea due to hypofunction of the spleen, fasting dysentery, metrorrhagia and leukorrhagia.

DIRECTIONS　To be eaten stewed, stir—fried or used as an ingredient of a prescription. It is used in most of tonifying medicated diet.

Quail Meat

ORIGIN　The meat or the whole substance, except the entralis and the feather, of Coturnix coturnix japonica, family Phasianidae.

NATURE, TASTE AND CHANNEL TROPISM　Sweet in taste, neutral in nature, and attributive to spleen, stomach and large intestine channels.

EFFICIENCIES　Tonifying the five viscera, clearing away damp—heat, arresting diarrhea and dysentery.

INDICATIONS　It is used for treatment of debility, diarrhea, dysentery, malnutrition of children due to impairment of the spleen and stomach, arthralgia of damp type.

DIRECTIONS　To be eaten stewed, stir—fried, deepfried, or decocted for drinking, or used as the main material of tonifying medicated diet.

Sparrow Meat

ORIGIN　The meat of the whole substance, except the entralis and the feather, of Passer montanus saturatus, family Ploceidae.

NATURE, TASTE AND CHANNEL TROPISM　Sweet in taste, warm in nature, and attributive to kidney and urinary bladder channels.

EFFICIENCIES　Strengthening yang, replenishing the vital essence, warming the loins and knees, and controlling urination.

INDICATIONS　It is used to treat magersucht due to yang deficiency, impotence, aching pain in the loins and knees, metrorrhagia and metrostaxis, leukorrhagia, frequent urination, hernia, etc.

DIRECTIONS To be eaten stir—fired, deep—fried, boiled, stewed or boiled down into soft extract.

Edible Bird's Nest

ORIGIN The nest built with saliva or saliva mixed with villus Collocalia esculenta ,family Apodidae, and many other swallows of the same breed.

NATURE, TASTE AND CHANNEL TROPISM Sweet in taste, neutral in nature, and attributive to lung, spleen and kidney channles.

EFFICIENCIES Nourishing yin to moisten dryness, tonifying qi and reinforcing the function of the spleen and stomach.

INDICATIONS It is used to treat consumptive diseases, tuberculosis, cough and phlegm—dyspnea, hemopthsis, hematemesis, protracted dysentery, chronic malaria, dysphagia and regurgitation.

DIRECTIONS To be boiled by putting the container in boiling water, or used to cook dishes or make medicated diet. It is to be soaked in warm water, cleaned of the feathers, blood and impure material before cooking.

Meat of Soft—Shelled Turtle

ORIGIN The meat of Amyda sinensis (Wiegmann), family Trionychidae.

NATURE, TASTE AND CHANNEL TROPISM Sweet in taste, neutral in nature, and attributive to liver channel.

EFFICIENCIES Nourishing yin and cooling the blood, restoring the vital energy and curing the diseases resulting from asthenia of viscera.

INDICATIONS It is used to treat consumptive fever due to yin deficiency, chronic malaria, protracted dysentery, metrorrhagia and metrostaxis, leukorrhagia, scrofula, weakness during convalescence, bodily weakness of the aged.

DIRECTIONS To be decocted in clear soup, steamed, or made into medicated diet. Pregnant women or those who manifest the syndrome of deificiency of yang of the spleen and stomach should avoid it.

SUPPLEMENT Turtle Shell: It is the back shell of the Chinese soft—

shelled turtle, Amyda sinensis(Wiegmann). Having the effects of nourishing yin to remove heat,calming the liver to relieve convulsion,softening the hard lumps, it is used to treat consumptive fever and hectic fever due to yin deficiency,convulsion due to deficiency of yin,malaria,mass in the abdomen,amenorrhea,metrorrhagia or metrostaxis,infantile convulsion. It is to be decocted or boiled down into soft extract for internal use,or used as an ingredient of boluses,pills or powder.

Section17

Astringents

This kind of drugs which are chiefly used to arrest or reduce excessive loss of the vital essence and body fluid are referred to as astringents of dietetic Chinese drugs.

Most drugs of this class are sour or astringent in flavour and have the effects of strengthening the superficial resistance to stop perspiration, astringing the bowels to arrest diarrhea, keeping the kidney essence, reducing urination, astringing the lung to relieve cough, and checking hemorrhage, curing leukorrhagia,etc. Astringents are indicated for syndromes of incessant and excssive loss of the body fluid or vital essence such as spontaneous sweating,night sweat,chronic diarrhea and dysentery, seminal emission, spermatorrhea, enuresis, frequent urination,chronic cough,asthma of insufficient type,metrorrhagia and metrostaxis, and protracted leukorrhagia due to general debility resulting from protracted illnesses and inconsolidation of the vital qi.

Astringents have the side effects of retaining the pathogenic factors so they should be avoided in cases of pathogenic factors of excess type.

Black Plam

ORIGIN Nearly riped fruit of Prunus mume (Sieb.) Sieb. et Zucc. ,family Rosaceae. Prepared by baking into black over slow fire.

NATURE, TASTE AND CHANNEL TROPISM　Sour and astringent in taste, warm in nature, and attributive to liver, spleen, lung and large intestine channels.

EFFICIENCIES　Astringe the intestine and relieve diarrhea; astringe the lung and relieve cough; promote the production of body fluid to quench thirst; calm the ascaris and alleviate pain; astringe and stop bleeding

INDICATIONS　1. For chronic diarrhea and cysentery with deficiency of healthy energy.

2. For prolonged cough and dry cough with weakness of vital energy.

3. For thirst due to yin—deficiency, or diabetes.

4. For abdominal pain caused by ascarides.

5. For hemafecia and metrorrhagia attributive to asthenia—syndrome. In addition, local application for callus and corn.

DIRECTION　Decoction: 3—10g.

Nutmeg

ORIGIN　Seed of Myristica fragrans Houtt., family Myristicaceae.

NATURE, TASTE AND CHANNEL TROPISM　Acrid in taste, warm in nature, and attributive to spleen, stomach and large intestine channels.

EFFICIENCIES　Astringe the intestine and relieve diarrhea, warm the middle—jiao and alleviate pain.

INDICATIONS　1. For prolonged diarrhea due to deficiency—cold of spleen and stomach, diarrhea before dawn due to deficiency—cold of spleen and kidney.

2. For stomach—cold with stagnation of vital energy manifested as abdominal pain, poor appetite and vomiting.

DIRECTIONS　Decoction: 3—10g.

Lotus Seed

ORIGIN　Seed of Nelumbo nucifera Gaertn., family Nymphaeaceae.

NATURE, TASTE AND CHANNEL TROPISM　Sweet and astringent

in taste, mild in nature, and attributive to spleen, kidney and heart channels.

EFFICIENCIES Benefit the kidney to preserve essence, keep the heart—fire and the kidney—water in balance, strengthen the spleen and relieve diarrhea, nourish heart and tranquilize the mind.

INDICATIONS 1. For diarrhea of spleen—deficiency type, palpitation, insomnia, amnesia, etc.

2. For nocturnal emission, enuresis and leucorrhagia attributive to kidney—deficiency. Also used for imbalance of the heart—fire and kidney—water manifested as nocturnal emission, palpitation, vexation, insomnia, dreaminess, tinnitus and soreness and weakness of the back and lower extremities.

DIRECTIONS Decoction: 9—18g, the embryo should be discarded when it is used as a tonic for invigorating the spleen and kidney, otherwise it should be retained.

Poria

ORIGIN The kernel of Euryale ferox Salisb, family Nymphaeaceae.

NATURE, TASTE CHANNEL TROPISM Sweet in taste, mild in nature, and attributive to spleen and kidney channels.

EFFICIENCIES 1. Strengthen the kidney to preserve essence, deprive dampness to relieve leucorrhagia.

2. Strengthen the spleen to relieve diarrhea.

INDICATIONS 1. For kidney—deficiency manifested as nocturnal emission, frequent micturition, enuresis, whitish and turbid urine, or leucorrhagia.

2. For diarrhea of spleen—deficieney type.

DIRECTION Decoction: 10—15g.

Chapter Three

Medicated Diet Treatment for Common Diseases and Syndromes

Section 1

Common Cold

Common cold is also known as "upper respiratory tract infection"; TCM holds that it results from exopathogens attacking the body. When having a cold, one can be treated with proper medicated diet according to the differentiation of syndromes so as to shorten the course of disease.

1. Common Types of Syndromes

1) Wind-Cold Type Manifested mainly as strong aversion to cold, slight fever without sweating, headache, stuffy nose, watery nasal discharge, itching of the throat, cough, expectoration of thin and white sputum, non-thirst or thirst and desire for hot drink, aching pain of limbs, thin and white fur, floating pulse or floating and tense pulse.

2) Wind-Heat Type Manifested as higher fever, light aversion to wind, slow sweat, distending pain in the head, stuffy nose , yellow and turbid nasal discharge, red-swollen and sore throat, or dry mouth and throat, thirst and strong desire for drink, cough, sticky or yellow phlegm, red margin and tip of the tongue with thin and white or light yellowish fur, floating and rapid pulse.

3) Summer-Heat and Dampness Type Manifested as catching cold in summer, marked by fever, light aversion to wind, absence of sweating or slight sweat, heaviness and distending pain in the head, vexation, thirst, heaviness sensation and aching pain of limbs, ropy and greasy mouth, thirst but drink little, oppressed sensation in the chest, nausea, oliguria with yellowish urine, thin and yellow fur or yellow and greasy fur, soft and floating and rapid pulse.

2. **Composite Medicated Diet**

1)Five-Ingredient Decoction(Wu Shen Tang)

INGREDIENTS

schizonepeta,Herba Schizonepetae 9g

clean perila leaf,Folium Perillae 9g

tea leaves,Folium Camelliae Sinensis 6g

fresh ginger,Rhizoma Zingiberis Recens 9g

brown sugar 30g

PROCESS Decoct the first four ingredients and sift the liquid from the dregs;then put in the brown sugar and stir it to have it dissolved.

DIRECTIONS To be taken in several separate doses on the same day. It is applicable to common cold of wind-cold type.

2)Drink of Mulberry Leaf,Chrysanthemum Flower,Peppermint and Prepared Soybean (Sang Ju Bo Chi Yin)

INGREDIENTS

mulberry leaf,Folium Mori 9g

chrysanthemum flower,Flos Chrysanthemi 9g

peppermint,Herba Menthae 6g

prepared soybean,Semen Sojae Praeparatum 6g

reed rhizome,Rhizoma Phragmitis 15g

(double the amount if fresh)

PROCESS Decoct them in water for oral administration. Or infuse them for drinking instead of tea.

DIRECTIONS The decoction is to be taken several times each day. It is applicable to common cold of wind-heat type.

3)Wrinkled Giant-Hyssop Drink (Huoxiang Dai Cha Yin)

INGREDIENTS

fresh leaves of wrinkled giant-hyssop,Folium Pogostemonis seu Agastachis 12g(reduce it to 6g if the dried is used)

fresh lotus leaf,Flium Nelumbinis 12g(6g if dried)

white sugar right amount

PROCESS Decoct them in water or infuse them in boiling water.

DIRECTIONS To be taken as a drink. It is applicable to those suffering from common cold of summer-heat and dampness type.

Section 2

Bronchitis

Bronchitis includes acute bronchitis and chronic bronchitis, both of which are mainly characterized by cough, expectoration and dyspnea. Acute bronchitis is characterized mainly by the types of wind-cold and wind-heat, chronic bronchitis can be divided into the types of phlegm-heat and deficiency of the lung. It belongs to the categories of "cough", "phlegm retention" and "asthma" in TCM.

1. **Common Types of Syndromes**

(1) The Type of Wind-Cold Marked by cough with itching of throat, thin and white expectoration, often accompanied with aversion to cold, fever without sweating, stuffy nose, watery nasal discharge, headache, aching pain in the limbs and so on, thin and whitish fur, floating or floating and tense pulse.

(2) The Type of Wind-Heat Marked by cough, dry and painful throat, difficult expectoration, ropy phlegm or thick and yellow phlegm, often accompanied with symptoms of aversion to wind, fever, thirst, perspiration, yellow nasal discharge, headache and so on, thin and yellow fur, floating and rapid pulse or floating and slippery pulse.

(3) The Type of Phlegm-Dampness Marked by cough, white and abundant phlegm which is ropy and greasy or thick, oppressed feeling in the chest and epigastric region, poor appetite, lassitude, white and greasy fur, soft and floating and slippery pulse.

(4) The Type of Phlegm-Heat Manifested as cough, abundant and yellow phlegm which is thick or ropy, dyspnea, oppressed feeling in the chest, fever, thirst, red tongue with yellowish and greasy fur, slippery and rapid pulse.

(5) The Type of Deficiency of the Lung Symptoms of frequent cough, shortness of breath, low voice, pale complexion, lassitude, pale tongue with thin and white fur, and thready and weak pulse attribute to deficiency of the lung-qi; while symptoms of frequent dry cough or cough with little or bloodtinged sputum, night sweat, dry mouth and throat, feverish sensation in the palms and

soles, or low fever, red tongue with thin fur, and thready and rapid pulse belong to deficiency of the lung-yin.

2. **Composite Medicated Diet**

1)Gruel of Perila Leaf and Apricot Kernel (Suye Xingren Zhou)

INGREDIENTS

perila leaf, Folium Perillae 9g

bitter apricot kernel, Semen Armeniacae Amarum 9g

tangerine peel, Pericarpium Citri Reticulatae 6g

Polished round-grained rice, Semen Oryzae Sativae 50g

PROCESS Decoct the first three ingredients in water, sift the liquid from the dregs, then put the rice in with a right amount of water and make them into gruel for eating.

INDICATIONS It is applicable to acute bronchitis of wind-cold type.

2)Drink of Chrysanthemum Flower and Apricot Kernel (Ju Xing Daicha Yin)

INGREDIENTS

chrysanthemum flower, Flos Chrysanthemi 6g

bitter apricot kernel, Semen Armeniacae Amarum 6g

mulberry leaf, Folium Mori 6g

liquorice, Radix Glycyrrhizae 3g

PROCESS Infuse all the ingredients in boiling water.

DIRECTIONS To be taken as a drink. It is suitable for acute bronchitis of wind-heat type.

3)Gruel of Two Chen and Two Kinds of Seeds(Erchen Erren Zhou)

INGREDIENTS

tangerine peel, Pericarpium Citri Reticulatae 9g

pinellia tuber, Rhizoma Pinelliae 6g

poria, Poria 12g

Job's tears seed, Semen Coicis 15g

shelled waxgourd seed, Semen Benincasae 15g

polished round-grained rice, Semen Oryzae Sativae 100g

PROCESS Decoct in water the first five ingredients, sift the decoction from the dregs; then put the rice into it with a right amount of water and cook them into gruel.

DIRECTIONS　To be taken in two separate doses each day. Applicable to patients suffering from chronic bronchitis of phlegm-dampness type.

4) Sichuan Fritillary Bulb and Pear Steamed with Additions (Fufang Chuanbei Li)

INGREDIENTS

Sichuan fritillary bulb, Bulbus Fritillariae Cirrhosae 6g

lily bulb, Bulbus Lilii 15g

water chestnut, Bulbus Heleocharis Tuberosae 30g

crystal sugar 15g

pear, Malun Piri 1 or 2

PROCESS　Steam all the ingredients together.

DIRECTIONS　The pear, water chestnut, lily bulb and juice are to be taken together. This recipe is applicable to chronic bronchitis of phlegm-heat type.

5) Gruel of Astragalus Root and Pork Lung (Huangqi Zhufei Zhou)

INGREDIENTS

pork lung (washed clean) 100g

astragalus root, Radix Astragali seu Hedysari 30g

polished round-grained rice, Semen Oryzae Sativae 100g

green Chinese onion, Bulbus Allii Fistulosi right amount

fresh ginger, Rhizoma Zingiberis Recens right amount

table salt right amount

gourmet powder right amount

PROCESS　First wash the pork lung clean, boil it in a right amount of water. When it is almost done, ladle it out and dice it for later use. Then decoct the astragalus root and remove the dregs. Put the rice and the diced pork lung into the decoction and make them into gruel. Finally season the gruel with the green Chinese onion, ginger, table salt and gourmet powder.

DIRECTIONS　To be taken in two separate doses each day. It is applicable to chronic bronchitis manifested as the type of insufficiency of the lung-yin.

6) Plain Spirits of Gecko with Additions (Fufang Gejie Jiu)

INGREDIENTS

gecko, Gecko (with no paws and head, and cut up) a pair

Chinese caterpillar fungus, Cordyceps 15g

astragalus root, Radix Astragali seu Hedysari 30g

plain spirits 1000g

PROCESS Soak the first three ingredients in plain spirits in a tightly sealed ceramic or glass container for 20 days. Sift the clear liquid at the upper part for drinking.

DIRECTIONS To be taken twice a day before meals, both in the morning and in the evening, 10 to 20 ml each time. The dregs can be re-used and soaked once more by adding a right amount of plain spirits to it. It is applicable to chronic bronchitis marked by the type of deficiency of both the lung and the kidney.

Section 3

Pneumonia

Pneumonia is classified according to pathologic anatomy into labor pneumonia, bronchial pneumonia and interstitial pneumonia. It is caused , as seen in Western medicine, by infection of bacteria, viruses or some other pathogen; while as seen in TCM, it results from pathogenic heat attacking the lung. It is marked mainly by cough, expectoration, dyspnea, oppressed feeling in the chest, and so on. Appropriate medicated diet can be selected as a supplementary treatment according to its syndromes at different stages.

1. **Common Type of Syndromes**

1) Wind-Heat Attacking the Lung Manifested at the initial stage of pneumonia as sudden invasion, aversion to cold or chills , fever, cough, non-productive cough with white and ropy sputum, oppressed feeling or dull pain in the chest, thirst, absence of sweating or hypoidrosis, red margin and tip of the tongue with thin and yellow fur, and floating and rapid pulse.

2) Excessive Accumulation of Lung-Heat Manifested as high fever, excess drinking due to thirst, serious cough, yellowish and thick expectoration, or cough with blood-stinged sputum or rusty sputum, rapid breathing , oppressed feeling and pain in the chest, flushed face or slight purple lips, red tongue with yellow fur, and slippery and rapid pulse.

3) Impairment of both Qi and yin Manifested at the restoration stage as

pyretolysis, mild cough, reduced expectoration. It is the impairment of the lung and yin if accompanied with dry mouth, vexation, slight fever, night sweat, red tongue, thready and rapid pulse; it is deficiency of the lung-qi if accompanied with shortness of breath, disinclination to talk, spontaneous perspiration and lassitude.

2. **Composite Medicated Diet**

1) Drink of Honeysuckle Flower and Chrysanthemum Flower with Additions (Fufang Yin Ju Cha)

INGREDIENTS

honeysuckle flower, flos Lonicerae 21g

chrysanthemum flower, Flos Chrysanthemi 9g

mulberry leaf, Folium Mori 9g

bitter apricot kernel, Semen Armeniacae Amarum 6g

reed rhizome, Rhizoma Phragmitis 30g

(double it if the fresh is used)

honey, Mel 30g

PROCESS Decoct the first five ingredients in water, discard the dregs and add honey to the decoction.

DIRECTIONS To be taken as a drink. Applicable to pneumonia at the initial stage marked by the syndrome of wind-heat attacking the lung.

2) Gruel of Reed Rhizome and Bamboo Juice (Lugen Zhuli Zhou)

INGREDIENTS

reed rhizome, Rhizoma Phragmitis 60g

(double it if the fresh is used)

polished round-grained rice, Semen Oryzae Sativae 50g

bamboo juice, Succus Bambusae 30g

crystal sugar 15g

PROCESS First decoct the reed rhizome in water, remove the dregs from the decoction; then put the rice into the decoction with a right amount of water and make gruel out of them. When the gruel is done, add in the bamboo juice and crystal sugar and go on cooking for a short while before it is ready for eating.

DIRECTIONS To be taken once or twice a day. Those who suffer from pneumonia manifested as the type of excessive accumulation of lung-heat can take it as an auxiliary treatment.

3) Five-Juice Drink (Wu ZHi Rin)

INGREDIENTS

juice of water chestnut, Bulbus Heleocharis Tuberosae

juice of fresh reed rhizome, Rhizoma Phragmitis Recens

juice of fresh lotus root, Rhizoma Nelumbinis Recens

juice of pear, Malum Piri

juice of lilyturf root, Radix Ophiopogonis

PROCESS Mix the same amount of all the five ingredients.

DIRECTIONS To be taken three times a day, 30ml each time. Applicable to patients suffering from pneumonia at the restoration stage marked by the type of impairment of the lung-yin manifested as lower fever, dry mouth and vexation.

Section 4

Bronchial Asthma

Bronchial Asthma (called asthma for short) is a common chronic disease that results from bronchospasm, mucocus edema and increasing secretion due to allergic reaction, and is clinically characterized by paroxysmal oppressed feeling in the chest, coughing, expiratory dyspnea and wheezing, even opening mouth and raising shoulders for breath, and even having difficulty in lying flat.

Asthma is called "wheezing syndrome" in TCM. Phlegm is thought as the major pathogenic factor of asthma in TCM. Whereas the disease may manifest itself in lung. Its origin can be traced to the spleen and kidney. Its principles of treatment call for a differentiation of evil and rightness, relief and urgence, and deficiency and excess in accordance with the process of the disease and the situation of attack.

Its medicated diet treatment can be selected and used in light of its clinical manifestations based on differential diagnosis.

1. **Common Types of Syndroms**

1) At the stage of attack, there are two types of syndromes, namely, asthma of cold type and asthma of heat type.

(1)Asthma of Cold Type Manifested as rapid breathing, wheezing sound in the throat, choking sensation in the chest much like asphyxia, dimmish and blackish complexion, cold extremities, non-thirst or thirst but desire for hot drink, easy to be attacked in cold weather or when taken with cold, white and slippery fur, wiry and tense pulse or floating and tense pulse.

(2)Asthma of Heat Type Marked by dyspnea and raucous breathing, thunderous rale in the throat, fits of irritated cough, cough with yellow, ropy and thick phlegm, difficult expectoration, vexation, restlessness, flushed face, bitter taste, thirst and desire for drink, perspiration, or accompanied with fever, red tongue with yellowish and greasy fur, slippery rapid pulse.

2)At remission stage, it is manifested in most cases as deficiency of the lung, spleen and kidney.

(1)Deficiency of the lung Manifested as catching common cold easily, shortness of breath, low voice, spontaneous perspiration, aversion to wind, asthma induced by any change of weather, pale tongue, thready and weak pulse.

(2)Deficiency of the Spleen Marked by poor appetite, fullness in the stomach at usual time, lassitude, loose stool, or diarrhea after eating greasy food, asthma often induced by improper diet, pale tongue, moderate and weak pulse.

(3)Deficiency of the Kidney Marked by shortness of breath at usual time which is characterized by inspiratory dyspnea, aggravated asthma due to exertion, susceptivity of asthma attack due to overwork, dizziness, tinnitus, lassitude in the loins and legs. In the case of those who indicate the syndrome of yang deficiency, it is marked by aversion to cold, cold limbs, thick and tender tongue; while in the case of those who show the syndrome of deficiency of yin, it is marked by feverish sensation in the palms and soles, vexation, flushing of zygomatic region, red tongue with little fur, thready and rapid pulse.

2. **Composite Medicated Diet**

1)Gruel of Ephedra and Dried Ginger (Mahuang Ganjiang Zhou)

INGREDIENTS

ephedra, Herba Ephedrae 6g

dried ginger, Rhizoma Zingiberis 6g

liquorice, Radix Glycyrrhizae 3g

polished round-grained rice, Semen Oryzae Sativae 100g

Chinese green onion, Bulbus Allii Fistulosi (cut up) 3g

PROCESS Decoct the first three ingredients and strain the dregs out from the decoction; then put the rice into the decoction with a right amount of water and make gruel. Finally when the gruel is done, scatter the cut-up Chinese green onion into it.

DIRECTIONS To be taken twice each day. It can be used as an auxiliary treatment for asthma of cold type.

2) Soft Extract of Sichuan Fritillary Bulb and Pear with Additions (Jiawei Beimu li Gao)

INGREDIENTS

Sichuan fritillary bulb, Bulbus Fritillariae Cirrhosae 30g
bitter apricot kernel, Semen Armeniacae Amarum 20g
root of purple-flowered peucedanum, Radix Peucedani 15g
gypsum, Gypsum Fibrosum 30g
licorice root, Radix Glycyrrhizae 10g
red tangerine peel, Exocarpium Citri Reticulatae 30g
snow pear, Pyrus nivalis 6
waxgourd, Fructus Benincasae 100g
crystal sugar 150g
alum, Alumen right amount

PROCESS First decoct in water the bitter apricot kernel, root of purple-flowered peucedanum, gyspum and raw licorice root and sift out 500ml of the decoction; cut the waxgourd strips into bits as small as soybeans, break the Sichuan fritillary bulb into pieces and grind the red tangerine peel into powder; peel and pound the pears and mix them with the alum solution. Then put into the solution the waxgourd bits, the scrumbs of the crystal sugar, the broken Sichuan fritillary bulb, the red tangerine peel powder. And then pour the decoction into them in a big bowl and mix them well. Finally put the bowl of the mixture in a food steamer and steam it with the bowl in the boiling water for about 50 minutes until it becomes sticky and thick extract.

DIRECTIONS To be taken in several days, in the amount which one thinks fit per day. Suitable for asthma of heat type.

3) Spirits of Ginseng Gecko and Cordyceps (Shen Ge Chong-cao Jiu)

INGREDIENTS

ginseng, Radix Ginseng 30g

cordyceps, Cordyceps 30g

walnut kernel, Semen Juglandis 30g

gecko, Gecko (with no head and paws) a pair

plani spirits 2000g

PROCESS Soak the first four ingredients in the 2000g of plain spirits in a tightly sealed ceramic or glass container for 20 days. Then sift the clear liquid at the upper part for drinking.

DIRECTIONS To be taken twice a day before meals, both in the morning and in the evening, 10 to 20 ml each time. The dregs can be re-used and soaked once more by adding a right amount of plain spirits to them. The spirits can tonify the lung and kidney, invigorate yang and yin, improve inspiration by invigorating the kidney and relieve asthma. Applicable to bronchial asthma at remission stage marked by the syndrome of deficiency of both the lung and the kidney.

4) Baby Pigeon Steamed with Ginseng, Astragalus Root and Cordyceps (Shen Qi Chongcao Ruge)

INGREDIENTS

ginseng, Radix Ginseng 3g (or dangshen, Radix Codonopsis Pilosulae 15g)

astragalus root, Radix Astragali seu Hedysari 15g

poria, Poria 15g

white atractylodes rhizome, Rhizoma Atractylodis Macrocephalae 9g

tangerine peel, Pericarpium Citri Reticulatae 6g

cordyceps, Cordyceps 6g

baby pigenon that has not moulted yet (get rid of its feathers and entrails)

PROCESS Place all the ingredients in a big bowl with a right amount of water; then steam them by putting the big bowl in boiling water in a food steamer, when the pigeon is welldone, season them with table salt and gourmet powder.

DIRECTIONS The pigeon is for eating and the soup for drinking. It is applicable to bronchial asthma at remission stage marked by deficiency of the lung, spleen and kidney.

Section 5

Acute and Chronic Enteritis

Acute and chronic enteritis can be both induced by kinds of causes of disease, but the main clinical manifestation of them is diarrhea, so they belong to "xie xie" in TCM. Appropriate medicated diet treatment can act as an auxiliary treatment or recuperation during the convalescence of the disease.

1. **Common Types of Syndromes**

1) Cold-Dampness (or Wind-Cold) Manifested as clear and thin, even watery diarrhea, abdominal pain, borborygmus, stuffiness in the stomach, poor appetite or accompanied with aversion to cold, fever, headache, stuffy nose, aching pain in limbs, thin and whitish fur or whitish and greasy fur, soft, floating and moderate pulse.

2) Damp-Heat (or Summer-Heat) Manifested as abdominal pain and diarrhea which is drastic, or accompanied with difficulty, yellow-brown and offensive feces, burning sensation at anus, dysphoria, thirst, dark urine, yellow and greasy fur, soft floating and rapid pulse or slippery and rapid pulse.

3) Deficiency of the Spleen Manifested sometimes as loose stool and at other times as diarrhea, presence of indigested food in the stool, more frequent stools after taking an irregular meal or a bit more greasy food, poor appetite, discomfort and stuffiness in the stomach after meals, lassitude, sallow complexion, pale tongue with whitish fur, thready and weak pulse.

4) Deficiency of the Kidney-yang Marked by abdominal pain before dawn, then borborygmus and diarrhea, feeling comfortable after diarrhea, cold sensation in the abdomen, cold limbs, lassitude in the loins and knees, pale tongue with whitish fur, deep and thready pulse.

2. **Composite Medicated Diet**

1) Gruel of Agastache and Roasted Ginger (Huoxiang Weijiang Zhou)

INGREDIENTS

agastache, Herba Pogostemonis seu Agastachis 6g

roasted ginger, Rhizoma Zingiberis Recens 6g

ledebouriella root, Radix Ledebouriellae 3g

round cardamon seed, Fructus Amomi Rotundus 3g

polished rond-grained rice, Semen Oryzae Sativae 100g

PROCESS Decoct the first four ingredients in water and remove the dregs from the decoction; then make gruel with the rice and a right amount of water. When the gruel is done, pour in the decoction and cook them for a few minutes.

DIRECTIONS To be taken hot so that the patient can perspire a bit, which will lead up to a best curative effect. It is applicable to diarrhea of cold-dampness type or wind-cold type.

2) Composite Drink of Lotus Leaf (Fufang Heye Cha)

INGREDIENTS

fresh lotus leaf, folium Nelumbinis Recens 6g

fresh lophatherum, Herba Lophatheri Recens 6g

fresh hyacinth-bean flower, Flos Dolichoris Recens 6g

fresh agastache, Herba Agastachis Recens 6g

PROCESS Decoct all of them in water.

DIRECTIONS To be taken as a drink. It is applicable to patients with diarrhea of damp-heat or summer-heat-dampness types.

3) Eight-Ingredient Cake (Ba Zhen Gao)

INGREDIENTS

Job's-tears seed, Semen Coicis 90g

euryale seed, Semen Euryales 90g

hyacinth bean, Semen Dolichoris Album 90g

lotus seed, Semen Nelumbinis 90g

Chinese yam, Rhizoma Dioscoreae 90g

dangshen, Radix Codonopsis Pilosulae 60g

poria, Poria 60g

white atractylodes rhizome, Rhizoma Atractylodis Macrocephalae 30g

white sugar 240g

PROCESS Grind the above ingredients into fine powder; them mix well the powder with the rice flour and water and make cakes by steaming the mixture.

DIRECTIONS To be taken any time as one wishes. The cake can be cut into pieces, toasted and stored for eating at ordinary times. This recipe, can replenish qi to invigorate the spleen and excrete dampness. It is very good for patients suffering from diarrhea due to chronic enteritis manifested as the type of deficiency of the spleen.

4) Gruel of Cherokee Rose-Hip (Jiawei Jinyingzi Zhou)

INGREDIENTS

cherokee rose-hip, Fructus Rosae Laevigatae 12g
baked ginger, Rhizoma Zingiberis Praeparata 6g
nutmeg, Semen Myristicae 6g
schisandra fruit, Fructus Schisandrae 3g
lotus seed, Semen Nelumbinis 15g
euryale seed, Semen Euryales 15g
Chinese yam, Rhizoma Dioscoreae 15g
polished round-grained rice, Semen Oryzae Sativae 50g

PROCESS Decoct the first four ingredients and remove the dregs from the decoction; then make gruel with the last four ingredients, the decoction and a right amount of water.

DIRECTIONS To be taken twice on the same day. Applicable to patients suffering from diarrhea due to chronic enteritis marked by the type of deficiency of the kidney-yang.

Section 6

Gastroduodenal Ulcers

Gastroduodenal ulcers is categorised as "epigastric pain", "acid regurgitation" or "distress in the stomach" in TCM. It rank in the list of common and frequently occurring internal diseases and mostly affected among adolescent or middle-aged patients. They are chronic in nature and often relapse. Clinically, their symptoms include periodic and rhythmic pain, accompanied by acid regurgitation, belching and vomiting etc.

Its pathogenic factors include deficiency and excessiveness, deficiency refers to the deficiency in the spleen and stomach, excessiveness refers to those pathogenic factors which irritate the stomach. The latter include catching cold, eating too much raw and cold food, or improper ingestion leading to food stagnancy, dyspepsia and endogenous damp-heat, and blocked Qi stemming from liver dysfunction and affecting stomach. Their cause of disease, treatment and recuperation during convalescence all have much to do with food and drink.

1. **Common Types of Syndromes**

1) The Pathogenic cold factor invades the stomach. It is manifested as sudden and violent stomachache, aggravated when the epigastrium is exposed to cold alleviated when it is warmed, desire for hot food and drink, thin and whitish fur, wiry and tense pulse.

2) Hepatic Qi affects the stomach   Manifested as distending pain in the stomach which radiates costal region and frequent eructation, which will get more serious whenever the patient is angry, thin and white fur, deep and wiry pulse.

3) Retention of food and drink in the stomach   It is marked by stomachache and fullness in the epigastrium, nausea, eructation with foul odour, acid regurgitation or vomiting of indigested food, relief of pain after vomiting, thick and greasy fur, slippery pulse.

4) Yin deficiency of the stomach   Manifested as dull stomachache, burning sensation in the stomach, dry mouth and throat, red and dry tongue, thready and rapid pulse.

5) Asthenia-cold in the spleen and stomach   Marked by dull pain in the stomach, desire for warmth and pressure over the affected part, extreme pain before meals, relief after meals, mental tiredness, poor appetite, loose stools, cold extremities in serious cases, pale tongue, deep and thready pulse or slow and moderate pulse.

6) Blood Stasis   Marked by stomachache so severe that the patient refuses to be pressed over the affected part, or as if the stomach were being pricked by needles, and the pain stays at the fixed region. It is manifested as hematemesis and melena if the condition gets more severe, and as purplish dark tongue or with ecchymoses, wiry and unsmooth pulse.

2. **Composite Medicated Diet**

1) Stomach-Warming Chicken (Nuan Wei Ji)

INGREDIENTS

roaster

fresh ginger, Rhizoma Zingiberis Recens 6g
amomum fruit, Fructus Amomi 3g
cloves, Flos Caryophylli 3g
galangal rhizome, Rhizoma Alpiniae Officinarum 3g
cassia bark, Cortex Cinnamomi 3g
tangerine peel, Pericarpium Citri Reticulatae 3g
long peper, Fructus Piperis Longi 3g
pricklyash peel, Pericarpium Zanthoxyli 3g
star anise fruit, Fructus Anisi Stellati 3g
green Chinese onion, Bulbus Allii Fistulosi, right amount
soy sauce and table salt right amount
pepper powder a little

PROCESS Skin the roaster, get rid of the entrails, wash it clean, cut it into pieces and put them in an earthenware pot with all the other ingredients but the pepper powder and a right amount of water; then stew it over slow fire, and when it is done, scatter the pepper powder on it.

DIRECTIONS The meat is for eating and the soup for drink. It is to be taken as much as one thinks it fit each time. It is used to treat stomachache of asthenia-cold type or stomach-cold type.

2) Gruel Activating Qi and Promoting Digestion (Xingqi Jianwei Zhou)

INGREDIENTS

amomum fruit, Fructus Amomi 3g
tangerine peel, Pericarpium Citri Reticulatae 6g
fruit of citron, Fructus Aurantii 6g
finger citron, Fructus Citri Sarcodactylis 6g
polished round-grained rice, Semen Oryzae Sativae 100g

PROCESS Decoct the first four ingredients, sift the decoction from the dregs; then put the rice into the decoction with a right amount of water and make them into gruel.

DIRECTIONS To be taken twice each day for treatment of stomachache marked by the types of stagnation of qi.

3) Three-Immortal Gruel with Additions (Jiawei Sanxian Zhou)

INGREDIENTS

medicated leaven, Massa Fermentata Medicinalis 12g

hawthorn fruit, Fructus Crataegi 12g

parched germinated barly, Fructus Hordei Germinatus Praeparatus 12g

Parched rice sprout, Fructus Oryzae Germinatus Praeparatus 12g

tangerine peel, Pericarpium Citri Reticulatae 6g

polished round-grained rice, Semen Oryzae Sativae 100g

PROCESS Decoct the first five ingredients in water, remove the dregs from the decoction; then add in the rice and a right amount of water and cook them into gruel.

DIRECTIONS To be taken twice each day. It is applicable to stomachache of indigestion type.

4) Egg Steamed with Notoginseng and Lotus Root Juice (Sanqi Ouzhi Dun Jidan)

INGREDIENTS

egg 1

fresh lotus root juice, Succus Rhizomatis Nelumbinis 30 ml

notoginseng powder, Pulvis Radicis Notoginseng 3g

PROCESS First beat the egg in a bowl, put in the other two ingredients and mix them well; then steam it by putting the bowl in boiling water in a pot.

DIRECTIONS To be taken once or twice a day. Applicable to patients suffering from stomachache of blood stasis type.

5) Drink of Fragrant Solomonseal Rhizome, Dendrobium, Black Plam and Hawthorn Fruit (Yu Shi Mei Zha Yin)

INGREDIENTS

fragrant solomonseal rhizome, Rhizoma Polygonati Odorati 6g

dendrobium, Herba Dendrobii 6g

hawthorn fruit, Fructus Crataegi 6g

white peony root, Radix Paeoniae Alba 6g

black plam, Fructus Mume 3g

liquorice, Radix Glycyrrhizae 3g

PROCESS Decoct in water all of the ingredients.

DIRECTIONS To be taken as a drink. It is applicable to stomachache marked by syndrome of deficiency of yin, and also good for atrophic gastritis marked by hypochlorhydria.

6) Pork Stomach Stewed with Pepper and Amomum Fruit (Hujiao Sharen

Dun Zhudu)

INGREDIENTS

pork stomach 1

black pepper, Fructus piperis Nigri 6g

amomum fruit, Fructus Amomi 6g

dried ginger, Rhizoma Zingiberis 6g

tangerine peel, pericarpium Citri Reticulatae 3g

cassia bark, Cortes Cinnamomi 3g

green Chinese onion, Bulbus Allii Fistulosi right amount

soy sauce and table salt right amount

PROCESS First wash the pork stomach clean, place it in an earthenware pot with a right amount of water, and add in all the ingredients; then stew it over slow fire until it is well-done.

DIRECTIONS To be taken as much as the patient thinks it fit. It is used to treat stomachache of stomach-cold type or asthenia-cold type.

Section 7

Hepatocirrhosis

Hepatocirrhosis (HC) is a chronic disease which affects the entire body. Its pathological features include degeneration, necrosis and regeneration of the hepatic cells; porliferation of hepatic fibrous tissue, and disturbance to the normal hepatic structure which lead to deformation and cirrhosis of the liver. Hence the term "hepatocirrhosis" comes into being. For the convenience of clinical observation and analysis of the state of illness, it can be classified into two stages: compensatory phase and decompensatory phase.

In TCM, it belongs to the categories of "Mass in the abdomen", "tympanites" etc. According to symptom-sign differentiation, it is ascribed to deficiency in the base and excessiveness in the superficies. It is often caused by the impairment of the liver, spleen and kidney, and the accumulation of Qi, blood and water. The general treatment regimen for HC calls for the elimination of blood stasis and the regulation of Qi, the softening of solids and the dissipation of mass, the excretion of dampness and the draining of water, and finally the attending to the improvement of patient's resistance. And Chinese medicated diet is usually used as an auxiliay treatment of hepatocirrhosis.

1. **Commom Types of Syndromes**

1)Compensatory Phase The common types of syndromes are as follows:

(1)Stagnation of Qi It is manifested as distending pain in the hypochondrium, which wanders up and down in this region with the pain having something to do with mood, accompanied with oppressed feeling in the chest, eructation, flatulence and so on , thin and white fur, wiry pulse.

(2)Blood Stasis Marked by twinge in the hypochondrium, which occurs in the fixed region, hematosplenomegaly, dark purplish tongue or with ecchymoses, deep and unsmooth pulse.

(3)Deficiency of the Spleen Manifested as lassitude, poor appetite, or loose stools, dropsy, pale tongue, thready and moderate pulse.

(4)Deficiency of Yin Marked by dull pain in the hypochondrium, dizziness, dry mouth and throat, vexation, feverish sensation in the palms and soles, lassitude in the loins and knees, insomnia, dreaminess, red tongue with little fur, thready, wiry and rapid pulse.

2)Decompensatory Phase The most conspicuous manifestation during this phase is ascitic fluid, which can be treated as "tympanites" on the basis of differentiation of syndromes in TCm. Tympanites is divided into tympanites due to stagnation of qi, ascites, and tympanites due to blood stasis.

(1)Tympanites due to Stagnation of Qi The abdomen distends so much as if it were a drum, but does not feel hard yet when pressed; it is sometimes large and sometimes small, sometimes mild and sometimmes severe; it is also manifested as fullness sensation in the chest and diaphragm, oliguria with painful urine, dysuria, wiry pulse.

(2)Ascites The abdomen is as large as a drum, and feels so full and solid when pressed as if it were a bag full of water; it gives out sounds when the patient is turnig over; or it is accompanied with dropsical extremities, oliguria, white and greasy fur, deep, wiry and slippery pulse.

(3)Tympanites due to Blood Stasis It is marked by abdomen as large as a drum, purple veins standing out, masses in the abdomen, emaciation, tawny complexion, drysuria, or melena, dark-purplish tongue or with ecchymoses, deep and wiry pulse or unsmooth pulse.

2. **Composite Medicated Diet**

1) Peach Kernel Gruel with Additions (Fufang Taoren Zhou)

INGREDIENTS

peach kernel, Semen Persicae 9g

tangerine peel, pericarpium Citri Reticulatae 6g

raw hawthorn fruit, Fructus Crataegi 12g

polished round-grained rice, Semen Oryzae Sativae 100g

PROCESS Decoct the first three ingredients in water, remove the dregs from the decoction; then add the rice and a right amount of water to the decoction and cook them into gruel.

DIRECTIONS To be taken twice each day for the treatment of early cirrhosis belonging to stagnation of qi and blood stasis.

2) Soup of Pork Stewed with Dangshen and Astragalus Root with Additions (Fufang Shen Qi Zhurou Tang)

INGREDIENTS

dangshen, Radix Codonopsis Pilosulae 12g

astragalus root, Radix Astragali seu hedysari 12g

poria, Poria 12g

white atractylodes rhizome, Rhizoma Atractylodis Macrocephalae 9g

lucid ganoderma, Ganoderma Lucidum 6g

tangerine peel, Pericarpium Citri Reticulatae 6g

finger citron, Fructus Citri Sarcodactylis 6g

amomum fruit, Fructus Amomi 3g

lean pork 100g

green Chinese onion, Bulbus Allii Fistulosi right amount

fresh ginger, Rhizoma Zingiberis Recens right amount

soy sauce and table salt right amount

PROCESS Stew the pork with all the ingredients and a right amount of water over slow fire until the pork is well-done.

DIRECRTIONS The meat is to be eaten and the soup to be drunk. It is applicable to patients suffering from early cirrhosis belonging to stagnation of the liver-qi and deficiency of the spleen.

3)Soup of Turtle Stewed with Chinese Angelica Root and Wolfberry Fruit (Gui Qi Jiayu Tang)

INGREDIENTS

Chinese angelica root, Radix Angelicae Sinensis 9g

wolfberry fruit, Fructus lycii 9g

prepared rehmannia rhizome, Radix Rehmanniae praeparata 6g

lilyturf root, Radix Ophiopogonis 6g

glossy privet fruit, Fructus Ligustri Lucidi 6g

Chinese yam, Rhizoma Dioscoreae 6g

tangerine peel, Pericarpium Citri Reticulatae 6g

turtle, Amyda Sinensis 1

green Chinese onion, Bulbus Allii Fistulosi right amount

fresh ginger, Rhizoma Zingiberis Recens right amount

PROCESS Put the first seven ingredients in a gauze bag; kill the turtle, cut it open, clean it of the entrails and wash it clean; place the gauze bag of drugs into the body cavity of the turtle, put the turtle in an earthenware pot, pour in a right amount of water and the seasonings. Stew the turtle with slow fire until it is well-done and then take out the bag of drugs.

DIRECTIONS The turtle is for eating and the soup for drinking. It is applicable to early cirrhosis manifested as the syndrome of deficiency of yin.

4)Gruel of Citron Fruit, Finger Citron and Radish Seed (Xiang Fo Laifu Zhou)

INGREDIENTS

citron fruit, Fructus Citri 9g

finger citron, Fructus Citri Sarcodactylis 9g

prepared radish seed, Semen Raphani (groud into powder) 15g

polished round-grained rice, Semen Oryzae Sativae 100g

PROCESS Decoct the first two ingredients in water, remove the dregs from the decoction; then add to the decoction the radish seed powder, the rice and a right amount of water and make them into gruel.

DIRECTIONS To be taken twice on the same day. Applicable to cirrhosis manifested as tympanites due to stagnation of qi.

5)Soup of Carp Inducing Diuresis (lishui Liyu Tang)

INGREDENTS

carp, Cyprinus Carpio 1 (about 250 to 500g)
corn stigma, Stigma Maydis 30g
red phaseolus bean, Semen Phaseoli 30g
waxgourd peel, exocarpium Benincasae 15g
poria, poria 15g
umbellate pore fungus, Polyporus 15g
rhizome of oriental water plantain, Rhizoma Alismatis 15g
tangerine peel, pericarpium Citri Reticulatae 6g
green Chinese onion, Bulbus Allii Fistulosi right amount
fresh ginger, Rhizoma Zingiberis Recens right amount

PROCESS First get rid of the scales of the carp, remove its entrails, wash it clean and place it in an earthenware pot; then put all the other ingredients into the pot with a right amount of water; after all this having been done, stew it with slow fire until the fish is well-done.

DIRECTONS The fish is to be eaten and the soup to be drunk. Applicable to ascites due to cirrhosis.

6) Gruel of Red Peony Root, Peach Kernel, Chinese Angelica Root and Poria (Chi Tao Gui Ling Zhou)

INGREDIENTS

red peony root, Radix Paeoniae Rubra 9g
peach kernel, semen persicae 9g
Chinese angelica root, Radix Angelicae Sinensis 9g
princesplume ladysthumb fruit, Fructus Polygoni Orientalis 6g
tangerine peel, Pericarpium Citri Reticulatae 6g
poria, Poria 12g
umbellate pore fungus, Polyporus 12g
red phaseolus bean, Semen Phaseoli 30g
polished round-grained rice, Semen Oryzae Sativae 60g

PROCESS Decoct the first seven ingredients in water, remove the dregs from the decoction; then add in the red phaseolus bean, the rice and a right amount of water and make them into gruel.

DIRECTIONS To be taken twice each day. applicable to cirrhosis manifested as the symptoms of tympanites due to blood stasis.

Section 8

Infantile Diarrhea

The main symptoms of this disease are marked by increased times of defecating, simultaneously accompanied with fever and mild vomiting, etc. Medicated dietetic therapy has a certain effect upon this disease.

1. **Common Types of Syndromes**

1) Impairment by overeating Marked by abdominal distention and pain, feces mixed up with indigested food which have a sour and fetid odor, abdominal pain ameliorated after the discharge of stools, accompanied with milk-mass vomiting, loss of appetite, sending out air with fetid odor, feverish sensation in the palms and soles, thick and greasy fur on the tongue, and slippery and rapid pulse.

2) Damp-heat Commonly seen in summer Marked by sudden onset of the disease, fever and vomiting, spouting diarrhea and tenesmus, watery feces usually with yellow—greenish colour, frequent diarrhea occuring more than ten times a day and with a sour and fetid odor, accompanied with irritability and thirst, scanty and yellowish urine, pale tongue with yellowish and greasy fur, and floating and rapid pulse.

3) Deficiency of the spleen Marked by diarrhea occuring several times a day, indigestion, thin and weak physique, sallow complexion, loss of appetite, sleeping with eyes half-closed, pale lips, pale and thick and tender tongue with little or thin and whitish fur, and thready, feeble pulse.

2. **Composite Recipes of Medicated Diet**

1) Gruel with Chicken's Gizzard-skin, Chinese Yam and Radish Seed (Neijin Shanyao Fuzi Zhou)

INGRDIENTS

radish seed, Semen Raphani 9g

chicken's gizzard-skin, Endothelium Corneum Gigeriae Galli 6g

Chinese yam, Rhizoma Dioscoreae right amount

white sugar right amount

PROCESS First, decoct the radish seeds and chicken's gizzard-skin in water to get extract; then put in the Chinese yam to make gruel. Mix it with white sugar and take it.

DIRECTIONS Children under the age of one year take about 10g at a time, the total gruel to be taken in two or three portions in one day; children above the age of one year can take as much as is thought fit. Take the drug for 3 to 5 days successively. It is applicable to the diarrhea due to impairment caused by overeating.

2) Recipe of Raw Coix Seed and Pulsatilla Root (Shengyimi Baitouweng Fang)

INGREDIENTS

raw coix seed, Semen Coicis 30g

pulsatilla root, Radix Pulsatillae 15g

husked sorghum, Semen Sorghi an appropriate amount

white sugar an appropriate amount

PROCESS Pop the husked sorghum in a pot and have 6g of it decocted in water together with raw coix seeds and pulsatilla roots to make decoction; add white sugar for oral administration.

DIRECTIONS A dose is to be taken in two or three separate portions a day for several days successively. It is applicable to the diarrhea of damp-heat type.

3) Decoction of Dangshen, Poria and Jujube (shen Ling Dazao Tang)

INGREDIENTS

dangshen, Radix Codonopsis Pilosulae 6g

poria, Poria 9g

Jujube, Fructus Ziziphi Jujubae 5pcs

roasted rice or millet 30g

brown sugar right amount

PROCESS Decoct the above ingredients in water to make decoction for oral administration.

DIERCTIONS Take a dose several times a day, for two or three days successively. It is applicable to the diarrhea of spleen-deficiency type.

Section 9

Enuresis in Children

This disease refers to the morbid state in which children over three years old unconsciously urinate in their sleep, realizing it only after waking up.

1. **Common Types of Syndromes**

1) Deficiency of the kidney-qi and kidney-yang Marked by frequent enuresis, yellowish pale complexion, cold hands and feet, the enuresis taking a turn for the worse in cold weather, lassitude in the loins and legs, light-coloured urine, pale tongue, and deep, thready and moderate pulse.

2) Failure in controlling urination due to deficiency of the spleen-qi and lung-qi Marked by frequent enuresis, pale complexion, weak limbs, spontaneous perspiration, loss of appetite, pale tongue with thin and white fur, and thready and weak pulse.

2. **Composite Recipes of Medicated Diet**

1) Recipe of Pork Urinary Bladder and Sophora Flower (Zhupangguang Huaihua Fang)

INGREDEIENTS

pork urinary bladder 1

sophora flower, Flos Sophorae 15g

dangshen, Radix Codonopsis Pilosulae 15g

PROCESS Have the pork urinary bladder cut open, washed clean and cut into cubes, and the sophora flowers and dangshen wrapped up with a piece of cloth; then put them into a pot and add water to cook them until the bladder is thoroughly done; remove the residues and take it after it's seasoned.

DIRECTIONS Take a dose every other day and take seven to eight doses in all. This recipe is applicable to the disease caused by deficiency of both the spleen-qi and lung-qi.

2) Recipe of Black Plum, Silkworm Cocoon and Jujube (Wumei Canjian Hongzao Fang)

INGREDIENTS

black (or green)plum, Fructus Mume 6g

silkworm cocoon, Coccum Bombycis 20g

jujube, Fructus Ziziphi Jujubea 10

white sugar 50g

PROCESS Make decoction for oral administration with the above ingredients.

DIRECTIONS Take it before four o'clock p. m. every day ,and that for days successively. It is applicable to the children who have the disease of the type with deficiency of the kidney—qi.

Section 10

Coronary Heart Disease

Coronary atherosclerotic heart disease, known as "coronary heart disease"or "coronary cardiopathy"for shot, is also called "ischemic heart disease". It refers to the heart disease induced by myocardial ischemia, and oxygen deficit caused by coronary atherosclerosis. In TCM, it pertains to the categories of "obstruction of Qi in the chest or in the heart". The mild case is named as"pectoral pains"; the serious case is named as"true heartache". This disease is located at the heart but is related to the spleen and the kidney. Its general mechanism is deficiency in the fundamental aspect of the body and excessiveness in the external symptoms. The fundamental aspect and external symptoms, deficiency and excess should be distingurshed when we differentiate types based on symptom-signs.

Mecicated diet therapy is both helpful and beneficial to the prevention, cure and recovery of this disease.

1. **Common Types of Syndromes**

1)Syndromes of Deficiency in Orgin The syndromes of deficiency of this disease include deficiency of qi, deficiency of yin and deficiency of yang

(1)Deficiency of the heart-qi Manifested as shortness of breath ,stuffiness in the chest, dyspnea due to exertion, lassitude, palpitation, disinclination to speak, perspiration, precordial dull pain, pale tonguewith teeth mark, weak , thready and relaxed pulse or irregular pulse.

(2)Deficiency of the heart-yin Marked by palpitation, vexation, insomnia, dizziness, dryness of mouth and throat, night sweat, precordial burning pain, reddened tongue, lack of saliva, little fur or without fur on the tongue, thready and rapid pulse.

(3)Deficiency of the heart-yang Characterized by aversion to cold, mental tiredness, shortness of breath, palpitation or severe palpitation, which is aggravated due to exertion, cold limbs, spontaneous perspiration, oppressed feeling in the chest, precordial pain which will be aggravated due to attack by cold, pale and bulgy tongue with white or greasy fur, weak, thready and slow pulse or irregular pulse.

2)Syndromes of Excess in Superficiality The syndromes of excess of this disease are divided into blood stasis, accumulation of phlegm, stagnation of qi, and accumulation of cold.

(1) Blood stasis Manifested as precordial twinge, colic, occuring in the fixed region and severe, accompanied with oppressed feeling in the chest for a long time if not cured, dark red or purplish dark tongue or tongue with ecchymoses, wiry and unsmooth pulse or irregular pulse.

(2) Accumulation of phlegm Marked by distinct oppressed feeling in the chest, accompanied with precordial pain, fat, vomiting with sputum or saliva in the vomitus, greasy fur, slippery pulse.

(3) Stagnation of qi Symptomatized by fullness and oppressed feeling in the chest, paroxysmal dull precordial pain, not occuring in the same region, desire for sighing , attack or aggravation due to unease of the mind, or accompanied with belch, distending pain in the hypochondria, fullness sensation in the stomach, thin and whitish fur, wiry or wiry and thready pulse.

(4) Accumulation of cold Manifested as sudden precordial pain so severe as if something twisted there, attack or aggravation after exposure to cold, cold hands and feet, perspiration with cold sensation, thin and white fur, and tense pulse.

2. **Composite Medicated Diet**

1)Drink of Peach Kernel and Hawthorn Fruit(Taoren Shanzha Daichayin)

INGREDIENTS

peach kernel, Semen Persicae 6g

hawthorn fruit, Fructus Crataegi 12g

tangerine peel pericarpium Citri Reticulatae 3g

PROCESS Infuse them in boiling water or decoct them in water.

DIRECTIONS To be taken as a drink. Applicable to patients suffering from coronary heart disease with obvious symptoms of blood stasis.

2) Gruel of Fleece-Flower Root and Lily Bulb (shouwu Baihe Zhou)

INGREDIENTS

prepared fleece-flower root, Radix polygoni Multiflori Praeparata 15to 30g

clean lily bulb, Bulbus lilii 30g

wolfberry fruit, Fructus Lycii 9g

Chinese-date, Fructus Ziziphi Jujubae 6pcs.

polished round-grained rice , Semen Oryzae Sativae 100g

white sugar right amount

PROCESS First decoct the first ingredient in an earthenware pot and sift thick liquid from the dregs; then make gruel out of the liquid and all the other ingredients.

DIRECTIONS To be taken both in the morning and in the evening. Applicable to patients suffering from coronary heart disease of yin deficiency type.

3) Gruel of Ginger, Bark of Chinese Cassia Tree and Masrostem Onion (Jiang Gui Xiebai Zhou)

INGREDIENTS

dried ginger, Rhizoma Zingiberis 3g

macrostem onion, Bulbus Allii Macrostemi 9g (double it if the fresh is used)

Chinese green onion, Bulbus Allii Fistulosi (which must be washed clean and cut up into small bits) 2

polished round-grained rice, Semen Oryzae sativae 100g

bark of Chinese Cassia tree powder , Pulvis Corticis Cinnamomi 0. 5to 1. 0g

PROCESS Make gruel with all the ingredients but the last one, when the gruel is done, scatter the powder of the bark of Chinese cassia tree over it.

DIRECTIONS To be taken once or twice per day. Applicable to patients suffering from coronary heart disease marked by the types of yang deficiency or accumulation of cold.

4) Soup of Seaweed and Laminaria (Haizao Kuenbu Tang)

INGREDIENTS

seaweed, Sargassum 30g

laminaria, Thallus Eckloniae 30g

jew's ear, Auricularia 15g

soybean, Semen Glycinis 200g

PROCESS Stew all the ingredients together, and when it is done, season it with a little amount of condiments.

DIRECTIONS For oral administration. Those who suffer from coronary heart disease complicated by hyperlipemia and hypertension can take it often.

5) Spirits of Ginseng, Red Sage Root and Hawthorn Fruit (Shuang Shen Shanzha Jiu)

INGREDIENTS

ginseng, Radix Ginseng 6g

red sage root, Radix Salviae Miltiorrhizae 30g

hawthorn fruit, Fructus Crataegi 30g

plain spirits 500g

PROCESS Soak the first three ingredients in the plain spirits in a bottle for 15 days.

DIRECTIONS To be taken twice or three times per day, 10 to 15ml each time. Applicable to patients suffering from coronary heart disease manifested as the types of deficiency of qi or blood stasis.

6) Honeyed Extract for Nourishing the Heart and Promoting Blood Flow (Yangxin Huoxue Migao)

INGREDIENTS

longan aril, Arillus longan 60g

mulberry, Fructus Mori 60g

lily bulb, Bulbus lilii 60g

poria with hostwood, Poria cum ligno Hospite 60g

wild jujuba seed, Semen Ziziphi Spinosae 60g

red sage root, Radix Salviae Miltiorrhizae 60g

hawthorn fruit, Fructus Crataegi 120g

safflower, Flos Carthami 30g

honey, Mel right amount

PROCESS Decoct all the ingredients except the last one three times; then put the three decoctions together to enrich them;finally make jelly by mixing the honey into the enriched decoction.

DIRECTIONS To be taken twice or three times per day, 20 to 30g each time. Those suffering from coronary heart disease with the manifestations of deficiency of the heart-qi, deficiency of the heart-yin, or blood stasis can take this honeyed jelly often.

Section 11

Congestive Heart-Failure

Congestive heart-failure refers to a series of clinical manifestations resulting from cardiac incompensation when an angiocardiopathy develops to a certain stage. According to its symptoms, it belongs to the categories of "palpitation", "severe palpitation", "dyspnea and cough", "phlegm retention"and "hydrops"

Medicated diet therapy can be used for the prevention and cure of light diseases, or for supplementary treatment of serious cases, or for nourishment during convalescence.

1. **Common Types of Syndromes**

1)Deficiency Syndrome It includes deficiency of qi, blood, yin and yang of the viscera, such as the heart, the spleen, the kidney and so on.

(1) Deficiency of the heart-qi Manifested as palpitation, shortness of breath, fatigue and weakness, dyspnea and suffocation due to exertion.

(2)Deficiency of the heart blood Manifested as palpitation, dizziness, lusterless complexion, lassitude and weakness, slightly pale tongue, thready and weak pulse.

(3)Deficiency of the heart-yin Manifested as palpitation, restlessness, vexation, insomnia, dizziness, red tongue with little fur or without fur, thready and rapid pulse.

(4)Deficiency of the heart-yang Manifedsted as palpitation, restlessness, oppressed feeling in the chest, shortness of breath, pale complexion, cold extremities, pale tongue, weak or deep, thready and rapid pulse.

(5)Deficiency of qi or blood is sure to be complicated by deficiency of the spleen;it is often the case that deficiency of yin has an influence on the liver and the kidney,while deficiency of yang affects the spleen and the kidney.

2)Excess Syndrome The excess syndromes of this disease are divided into blood stasis,turbid phlegm and excessive fluid.

(1)Excessive fluid Manifested as palpitation,vertigo,feeling of fullness in the chest and abdomen,cold extremities,oliguria,or edema of lower limbs,nausea,vomiting,salivation,white and greasy fur,wiry and slippery pulse.

(2)Turbid phlegm Manifested as palpitation,shortness of breath,feeling of fullness in the chest,adundant expectoration,poor appetite and fullness of sensation in the abdomen,or nausea,white and greasy or slippery and greasy fur, wiry and slippery pulse.

(3)Blood stasis Manifested as palpitation,restlessness,discomfort and oppressed feeling in the chest,frequent attack of precordial pain,or dark-purple lips and nails purple and dark tongue or tongue with ecchymoses or petechia,unsmooth or irregular pulse.

It is common that a patient has deficency syndrome and excess syndrome at the same time,which leads up to the coexistence of syndromse of deficiency in origin and syndromes of excess in superficiality,or the coexistence of deficiency and excess.

2. **Composite Medicated Diet**

1)Gruel of Longan Aril and Lily Bulb(Yuanrou Baihe Zhou)

INGREDIENTS

longan aril,Arillus Longan 15 to 30g

lily bulb,Bulbus Lilii 15 to 30g

Chinese-date,Fructus Ziziphi Jujubae 6pieces

polished round-grained rice,Semen Oryzae Sativae 100g

white sugar right amount

PROCESS Make gruel with them all.

DIRECTIONS To be taken both in the morning and in the evening.

INDICATIONS Applicable to those who suffer from congestive heart-failure with syndromes of deficiency of qi,yin and blood which are marked by frequent palpitation and shortness of breath.

2)Honeyed Extract of American Ginseng for Nourishing the Heart (Yang-shen Yixin Migao)

INGREDIENTS

root of American ginseng, Radix Panacis Quinquefolii 30g

ophiopogon root, Radix Ophiopogonis 150g

longan aril, Arillus Longan 250g

parched wild jujuba seed, Semen Ziziphi Spinosae 120g

PROCESS First decoct the four ingredients together three times; then put the three decoctions together and enrich the mixture to make extract, finally honey the extract.

DIRECTIONS To be taken twice a day , both in the mornig and in the evening 15 to 30g each time. Applicable to patients with syndrome of deficiency of the heart-yin manifested as palpitation, vexation, insomnia, dreaminess, dry mouth and throat.

3) Ginseng Decoction for Nourishing the Hreat (Renshen Yangxin Cha)

INGREDIENTS

ginseng, Radix Ginseng 3g

parched wild jujuba seed, Semen ZIziphi Spinosae 15g

poria with hostwood, poria cum Ligno Hospite 9g

tangerine peel , Percarpium Citri Reticulatae 3g

PROCESS Decoct them or infuse them in boiling water.

DIRECTIONS To be taken as a drink. Applicable to patients with syndrome of deficiency of the heart-yang manifested as palpitation, shortness of breath, fatigue and weakness.

4) Gruel of Cinnamon Twig, Dried Ginger and Ginseng (Gui Jiang Renshen Zhou)

INGREDIENTS

cinnamon twing, Ramulus Cinnamomi 6g

dried ginger, Rhizoma Zingiberis 6g

ginseng Radix Ginseng 3g

Chinese-date, Fructus Ziziphi Jujubae 8pieces

polished round-grained rice, Semen Oryzae Sativae 100g

brown sugar rightamount

PORCESS Decoct the first four ingredients together, when the water comes to the boil, decoct them with slow fire until they become thick juice; then cook the juice with rice and brown sugar until the gruel is done.

DIRECTIONS To be taken twice, both in the morning and in the evening. It is applicable to patients with syndrome of deficiency of the heart-yang manifested as palpitation, shortness of breath, mental tiredness, fatigue and cold extremities.

5) Quick-Dissolvable Drink of Fragrant Solomonseal Rhizome (Yuzhu Suring Yin)

INGREDIENTS

clean fragrant solomonseal rhizome, Rhizoma Polygonati Odorati 250g

dry white sugar powder 300g

PROCESS First soak in cold water fragrant solomonseal rhizome and, after it has become saturated and some more water has been added, decoct it three times, twenty minutes each time; then mix the three decoctions into one and continue decocting it over a slow fire until it is almost boiled away; and then, when it becomes warm, put in dry white sugar powder and mix them up to absorb all the decoction left; finally dry the mixture in the sun, grind the mixture and put it in a bottle for future use.

DIRECTIONS To be taken infused in boiling water, 3 times a day, 10g each time. Applicable to patients suffering from ordinary chronic heart-failure. Fragrant solomonseal rhizome can invigorate yin, moisten dryness, promote the production of body fluid and quench thirst. Modern study has shown that fragrant solomonseal rhizome contains cardiac glucyoside (convallamain, convallarin), and experiments on animals have proved that it has the functions of invigorating the heart, reducing blood sugar and actions similar to adrenocortical hormone, and clinical application proves that it is effective for congestive heart failure resulting from rheumatic heart disease, coronary heart disease or pulmonary heart disease. Thiis prescription is more applicable to patients suffering from heart failure marked by the type of deficiency of yin

6) Fragrant Solomonseal Rhizome and Pork Heart (Yuzhu Zhuxin)

MAIN INGREDIENTS

pork heart 500g

fragrant solomonseal rhizome, Rhizoma Polygonati Odorati 20g

SUBSIDIARY INGREDIENTS

canned water chestnut, Bulbusa Heleochais Tuberosae 50g

hotbed chives, Herba Allii Tuberosi 10g
chicken broth 40g
CONDIMENTS
refined salt 2. 5g
soy sauce 15g
cooking wine 10g
green Chinses onion, Allium Fistulosum 6g
fresh ginger, Rhizoma Zingiberis Recens 6g
watered starch 15g
sesame-seed oil, Oleum Sesami 15g
vegetable oil 500g (only 50g of it will be used up)
white sugar, peper powder and vinegar right amount

PROCESS Wash fragrant solomonseal rhizome clean, cut them into pieces, and decoct them in water three times; mix the three decoctions into one and enrich the mixture by boiling it until zoml of it is left. Slice up the pork heart, put the slices in a bowl and mix them with refined salt and watered starch. Wash the hotbed chives clean, cut them into 3-cm-long sections; slice up water chestnut, cut green Chinese onion, ginger and garlic into small bits. Place in a small seasoning bowl the cooking wine, soy sauce, white sugar, gourmet powder and refined salt; make thick liquid mixture of the peper powder, chichen soup, watered starch and the enriched fragrant solomonseal rhizome decoction for later use. After all this having been done, place a boiler over a fire pour in vegetable oil and put in the pork heart pieces to saute them; when they are well-done, pour them in a strainer to drain the oil. Put the boiler over the fire again, and when the remaining oil becomes hot, put in , first of all , the garlic bits, then the bits of green Chinese onion and ginger; fry them until a sweet smell comes off and put them in the sliced water chestnut; when it is well-done, put in the sauteed pork heart, followed by the thick liquid mixture, hotbed chive sections, and stir-fry them until they are done. Finally, drip in vinegar, a little sesame seed oil, and place them in a dish.

This diet has the functions of nourishing yin and blood, and tranquilizing the mind. It is applicable to patients suffering from deficiency of the heart-yin and deficiency of the heart-blood manifested as palpitation, vexation, insomnia and dreaminess, or deficiency of the lung-yin manifested as dry cough, chronic cough, or deficiency of the stomach-yin manifested as excessive thirst, loss of appetite and so on. It can also be used as cooked dishes for health care of patients suffering from chronic heart-failure.

Section 12

Essential Hypertension

Essential hypertension is a frequently seen disorder of cardiovascular system.

In TCM, it belongs to the categories of dizziness and headache. Its general mechanisms are"flaming-up of liver-fire, deficiency of both the liver-yin and the kidney-yin, and hyperactivity of yang due to yin deficiency.

Medicated diet can be used not only as a supplementary treatment for essential hypertension but also for its prevention and recovery and for health care.

1. **Common Types of Syndromes**

1) Flaming-up of Liver-fire It is mainly manifested as distending pain in the head, dizziness, flushed face, conjunctivel congestion, impetuosity and liability to anger, bitter taste, dry throat or accompanied with tinnitus, deafness, vexation, insomnia, which are aggravated by anger or overstrain, red tongue with yellow fur, wiry and rapid pulse.

2) Deficiency of both the Liver-yin and the Kidney -yin This type of syndrome is mainly manifested as dizziness, headache, dim eyesight, tinnitus, dry mouth, dryness in the eye, insomnia, dreaminess, feverish sensation in the palms and soles, lassitude in the loins and knees, mental tiredness, amnesia, red tongue with little fur, thready and wiry pulse or thready , wiry and rapid pulse.

3) Hyperacitivity of Yang due to Yin deficiency The syndrome of this type is marked by more serious distending pain in the head, occasionally flushed face, impetuosity and liability to anger, vexatiom, red tongue with thin and yellow fur, wiry, thready and rapid pulse as well as the symptoms of syndrome of deficiency of both the liver-yin and the kidney-yin.

2. **Composite Medicated Diet**

1) Drink of Hawthorn Fruit and Chrysanthemum Flower (Shanzha Juhau Daicha Yin)

INGREDIENTS

hawthorn fruit, Fructus Crataegi 12g

chrysanthemum flower, Flos Chrysantemi 9g

PROCESS Infuse them in boiling water for drinking.

DIRECTIONS Patients with essential hypertension or accompanied with hyperlipemia, coronary heart disease can take it regularly as tea; while those with essential hypertension marked by the types of liver-fire or hyperactivity of yang due to yin deficiency can take it as a supplementary medicine.

2) Thick Soup of Water Chestnut and Jellyfish Head (Xue geng Tang)

INGREDIENTS

water chestnut, Bulbus Heleochâris Tuberosae 100 to 200g

jellyfish head, Rhopilema 100 to 200g

PROCESS Cook soup with them.

DIRECTIONS To be taken twice or three times a day for the treatment of essential hypertension accompanied with syndrome of accumulation of phlegm manifested clinically as vertigo, heaviness sensation in the head, fullness and stuffiness in the chest and stomach, or vomiting, nausea, salivation, white and greasy fur, wiry and slippery pulse.

3) Soup of Corn Stigma and Tortoise (Yumixu Gui Tang)

INGREDIENTS

tortoise, Chinemys Reevesii (over 500g)

corn stigma, Stigma Maydis 120g

PROCESS Place the tortoise in a basin, pour in hot water; after the tortoise has discharged all its urine, wash it clean and cut off its head and feet, rid of its internal organs; then put it in an earthenware pot together with the corn stigma and a right amount of water. Cook on a strong fire until the water comes to the boil and then cook on with a slow fire until the torroise is well-done.

DIRECTIONS The flesh of the tortoise is for eating and the soup for drinking. It is used to treat essential hypertension manifested as the type of deficiency of both the liver-yin and the kidney-yin.

4) Gruel of Chrysanthemum Flower and Hawthorn Fruit (Juhua Shanzha Zhou)

INGREDIENTS

dried chrysanthemun flower, Flos Chrysanthemi (with no bases) 9 to 12g

hawthorn fruit slices, Fructus Crataegi 9 to 12g

polished round-grained rice, Semen Oryzae Sativae 45 to 60g

crystal sugar right amount

PROCESS Grind the first two ingredients into powder; then make gruel out of the rice, sugar and 500ml of water, when the rice begins to boil with the liquid not thick yet, mix the powder of the first two ingredients into the gruel and go on cooking on a slow fire for a while; and finally when the gruel becomes thick, put out the fire and simmer it for five minutes with the pot tightly covered.

DIRECTIONS To be taken warm, once or twice a day, for patients with essential hypertension or that accompanied with hyperlipemia, coronary heart disease. Stop taking it in winter.

Select one or two from among the recipes above that are to your taste. If curative, they should be taken for a long time.

Section 13

Chronic Hypotension

Chronic hypotension is manifested as various kinds of symptoms and signs, which are known in TCM as vertigo, deficiency syndrome and so on.

1. **Common Types of Syndromes**

1) Deficiency of both Qi and Yin Marked by dizziness, lassitude, palpitation, vexation, shortness of breath, dry mouth and throat, red tongue, thready pulse in most cases.

2) Deficiency of both Qi and Yang Marked by dizziness, lassitude, shortness of breath, mental tiredness, aversion to cold, spontaneous perspiration, palpitation, oppressed feeling in the chest, cold limbs, slightly pale and enlarged tongue, weak, thready and slow pulse.

2. **Composite Medicated Diet**

1) Pork Heart Stewed whit Dangshen and Cassia Twig (Shen Gui Dun Zhuxin)

INGREDIENTS

pork heart 1

dangshen, Radix Codonopsis Pilosulae 15g

astragalus root, Radix Astragali sea Hedysari 15g

bark of Chinese cassia tree, Cortex Cinnamomi 6g

cinnamon twig, Ramulus Cinnamomi 6g

Chinese angelica root, Radix Angelicae Sinensis 12g

tangerine peel, Pericarpium Citri Reticulatae 9g

liquorice, Radix Glycyrrhizae 9g

green Chinese onion, Allium Fistulosum right amount

fresh ginger, Rhizoma Zingiberis Recens right amount

table salt right amount

PROCESS First wash the pork heart clean and slice it up, put the slices in an earthenware pot, and pour in a right amount of water; then put in all the other ingredients; stew them over slow fire, and when the pork heart is well-done, discard the dregs.

DIRECTIONS The pork heart is to be eaten and the soup to be drunk. It is applicable to those who suffer from chronic hypotension manifested as deficiency of both qi and yang.

2) Gruel of Ginseng and Lilyturf Root with Additions (Jiawei Shengmai Zhou)

INGREDIENTS

ginseng, Radix Ginseng 6g

(or dangshen, Radix Codonopsis Pilosulae) 21g

lilyturf root, Radix Ophiopogonis 15g

Siberian solomonseal rhizome, Rhizoma Polygonati 15g

tangerine peel, Pericarpium Citri Reticulatae 12g

prepared liquorice, Radix Clycyrrhizae Praeparata 9g

schisandra fruit, Fructus Schisandrae 6g

polished round-grained rice, Semen Oryzae Sativae 100g

PROCESS First decoct in water all the ingredients but the rice and get the decoction by removing the dregs; then make gruel with the decoction, the rice and right amount of water.

DIRECTIONS To be taken twice each day . It is applicable to patients suffering from chronic hypotension marked by syndrome of deficiency of both qi and yin.

Section 14

Chronic Nephritis

chronic nephritis is clinically characterized by edema, proteinuria and hypertension. It in most cases falls into the categories of "Zheng shui"(anasarce with shortness of breath), "shi shui"(stony edema) and "yin shui"(yin-type edema). Medicated diet, as an auxiliary treatment, has a positive effect on both the improvement of symptoms of the disease and the recovery of the organism.

1. Common Types of Syndromes

1) Overflow of Water in the Body due to Insufficiency of both the Spleen-yang and the Kidney-yang Manifested as pale or sallow complexion, heavy edema of the whole body, abdominal distention so severe as if the abdomen were a drum, cool limbs and aversion to cold, poor appetite, loose stools, oliguria, light-colored urine, aching pain in the waist, pale but corpulent tongue with teeth marks on its margin, thin and white fur, deep and thready pulse or deep and slow pulse.

2) Insufficiency of both the Spleen and the Kidney with Deficiency of Essence and Blood Manitested as pale and lusterless complexion, mental and bodily tiredness, lassitude in the loins and knees, albuminuria, pale tongue, weak pulse.

3) Hyperactivity of the Liver-yang due to Deficiency of both the Liver-yin and the Kidney-yin Marked by dizziness, headache, poor vision, tinnitus, dysphorria with feverish sensation in the chest, palms and soles, dry mouth, desire for drinking water, restlessness in sleeping, lassitude in the loins and legs, red tongue with white fur, wiry, thready and rapid pulse.

2. Composite Medicated Diet

1) Egg Steamed with pepper (Hujiao Jidan)

INGREDIENTS

white pepper, Fructus Piperis Albi 7 grains

egg 1

PROCESS Make a small hole in the egg, put the seven grains of white pepper into it, seal the hole with flour and wrap the egg with wet paper. Then stam it in a food steamer until it is done.

DIRECTIONS The egg and the pepper are to be taken together after the egg is shelled, two eggs per day for adults, one for children, ten days making up one course of treatment. The second course of treatment is to begin following a suspension of three days.

It is used to treat chronic nephritis manifested as the type of insufficiency of both the spleen and the kidney with deficiency of essence and blood.

2)Thick Crucian Carp Soup (Jiyu Geng)

INGREDIENTS

big crucian carp, carassius Auratus 500g

garlic, Bulbus Allii 1

black pepper, Fructus Piperis Nigri 3g

pricklyash peel, Pericarpium Zanthoxyli 3g

tangerine peel, Pericarpium Citri Reticulatae 3g

amomum fruit, Fructus Amomi 3g

long pepper, Fructus Piperis Longi 3g

green Chinese onion, Bulbus Allii Fistulosi

thick sauce made from soybean

table salt

PROCESS Put all the other ingredients into the belly of the fish, and cook it; then make thick soup with it.

DIRECTIONS To be taken after seasoned. Applicable to chronic nephritis of all types.

3) Honeyed Prepared Rhizome of Rehmannia and Chinese Yam (Shudi Shanyao Mi)

INGREDIENTS

prepared rhizome of rehmannia, Radix Rehmanniae praeparata 60g

Chinese yam, Rhizoma Dioscoreae 60g

honey Mel 500g

PROCESS Wash the first two ingredients clean quickly, place them in an earthenware pot. pour in three big bowls of water, decoct them over slow fire for forty minutes and get a half bowl of the decoction; then add another bowl of cold water to the remaining drug, decoct them for thirty minutes until half bowl of the decoction is left and sift it out, mix the two half bowls of decoction with the 500g of honey, pour the mixture into a ceramic basin, cover it so as not to let any stam get into the basin. Finally steam it with strong fire for two hours, and when it becomes cool, put it into a bottle and cover it tightly.

DIRECTIONS To be taken after meals with warm boiled water, twice a day, one spoonful each time. Those who are debilitated due to chronic nephritis can take it as nourishment.

Section 15

Urinary Infection

Urinary infection, including pyelonephritis, cystitis and urethritis, is characterized clinically by lumbago, frequence and urgency of micturition, and urodynia. It belongs to "Linzheng"(stranguria) in TCM.

1. **Common Types of Syndromes**

1) Damp-heat of the Lower-jiao with Retention of Toxic Material in the Urinary Bladder Manifested as frequence and urgency of micturition, urethralgia, ascheturesis, abdominal distention, nausea or vomiting, poor appetite, thirst but no desire for drinking water, or afternoon low-grade fever, turbid and yellow urine, red tongue with yellow and greasy fur, slippery and rapid pulse.

2) Insufficiency of both the Spleen and Kidney with Retention of Toxic Material in the Lower-jiao Manifested as frequent micturition after overwork, no obvious urodynia and burning sensation of urethra. Urinary infection marked by insufficiency of the spleen is manifested as palpebral edema, swelling of the lower extremities, poor appetite, indigestion, loose stool, corpulent tongue with teeth marks on its margin, deep and moderate pulse; while that marked by insufficiency

of the kidney manifested as dizziness, insomnia, dreaminess, pain in the waist, lassitude in the lower extremities, emaciated and pale tongue, deep and thready pulse.

2. **Composite Medicated Diet**

1) Mung Bean Gruel (Qingxiaodou Zhou)

INGREDIENTS

mung bean, Semen Phaseoli Radiati 50g

ricepaper pith, Medulla Tetrapanacis 10g

Wheat, Fructus Tritici 50g

PROCESS First decoct the ricepaper pith in 2000ml of water and sift out 1000ml of the decoction; then make gruel with the 1000ml of decotion, the mung bean and the wheat for eating.

DIRECTIONS To be taken before meals. It can be used to treat urinary infection of the type of insufficiency of both the spleen and the kidney with retention of toxic material in the lower-jiao.

2) Tale Gruel (Huashi Zhou)

INGREDIENTS

tale Tacum (wrapped in a piece of cloth) 20 to 30g

Chinese pink herb, Herba Dianthi 10g

polished round-grained rice, Semen Oryzae Sativae 50 to 100g

PROCESS First decoct the first two ingredients in an earthenware pot and remove the dregs, and then add the rice to the decoction and make gruel with them.

DIRECTIONS This recipe can be widely used to treat acute uriary tract infection manifested as all the types. Pregnant women should avoid it.

It also can be chosen to treat urinary infection manifested as the type of damp-heat of the lower-jiao with retention of toxic material in the urinary bladder.

Section 16

Impotence

This symptom is manifested as inability to have an erection of the penis or lack of copulative power in males. According to the theory that kidney is the organ to make the penis erect, TCM considers it in most cases as insufficiency of the kidney-yang, therefore the drugs having the functions of reinforcing the kidney and strengthening the yang are chosen to treat it so as to promote its recovery. Medicated diet has a better curative effect on impotence.

1. **Common Types of Syndrome**

Insufficiency of the Kidney-yang   Manifested as impotence, dizziness, tinnitus, soreness in the loins and knees, lusterless complexion, listlessness, pale tongue with thin white fur, deep and thready pulse.

2. **Composite Medicated Diet**

1) Sea Cucumber and Mutton Soup (Haishen Yangrou Tang)

INGREDIENTS

sea cucumber, Stichopus Japonicus (cubed) 250g

mutton (cubed) 250g

fresh ginger, Rhizoma Zingiberis Recens

table salt

PROCESS   Stew the first two ingredients together.

DIRECTIONS   Season it with fresh ginger and table salt before it is eaten.

2) Gecko and Psoralea Fruit Powder (Gejie Buguzhi Fen)

INGREDIENTS

gecko, Gecko a pair

psoralea fruit, Fructus Psoraleae 25g

alcoholic drink

PROCESS   Stir-fry the geckoes in alcoholic drink and dry them over a fire, and then grind the geckoes and the psoralea fruit into fine powder.

DIRECTIONS   To be taken with warm alcoholic drink, 1.5g each time.

3) Epimedium Spirits (Xianlingpi jiu)

INGREDIENTS

epimedium, Herba Epimedii 60g

plain spirits 500ml

PROCESS   Fill a gauze bag with epimedium, soak it in plain spirits and seal the container. It can be taken after it has been soaked for three days.

DIRECTIONS To be taken at bedtime, 10 to 15 ml each time.

All the recipes above can reinforce the kidney and strengthen yang. Patients with impotence can choose one or two from among them regular eating according to the state of their illness.

Section 17

Seminal Emission

Seminal emission refers to spontaneous discharge of sperm not resulting from sexual intercourse. Medicated diet, as a supplementary treatment, has a certain curative effect on this symptom.

1. **Common Types of Syndromes**

1) Unconsolidation due to Kidney Deficiency Marked by frequent seminal emission, which takes place in most cases when the patient is dreamless, even spermatorrhea, accompanied with lassitude in the loins and legs, dizziness, tinnitus, pale tongue with white fur, deep and weak pulse.

2) Hyperactivity of Fire due to Yin Deficiency Manifested as frequent emission, aversion to heat, restlessness, feverish sensation in palms and soles, flushed face, red margin and tip of the tongue, thready and rapid pulse.

2. **Composite Medicated Diet**

1) Powder of Soft-Shelled Turtle's Head and Taill (jiayu Shou Wei San)

INGREDIENTS

the head and the tail of a newly-killed soft-shelled turtle, Trionyx Sinensii

sesame-seed oil, Oleum Sesami

PROCESS Deep-fry in sesame-seed oil the head and the tail of a newly-killed soft-shelled turtle until they are scorched, and then grind them respectively into powder.

DIRECTIONS Mix the powder of the head of the turtle into food and take it all before the meal. When recovered from the illness 100 days later, take the powder of the tail of the turtle the same way as you did with that of the head. The powder of the head of the turtle having been taken, the penis may become impotent, not erect any more, and you will not have the desire for sexuality and the phenomena of nocturnal emission and seminal emission will come to an end. It is not until 100 days or more (no less than those) later when the powder of the turtle's tail is taken that the penis will resume its original shape and the desire for sexuality will gradually become normal. Nevertheless, temperance in sexual life must be pracitised. This recipe is applicable to patients with seminal emission marked by the type of hyperactivity of fire due to yin deficiency.

2) Decoction of Oyster Shell, Rhizome of Wind-Weed and Lotus Seed (muli Zhimu Lianzi Tang)

INGREDIENTS

raw oyster shell, Concha Ostreae 20g

rhizome of wind-weed, Rhizoma Anemarrhenae 6g

lotus seed, Semen Nelumbinis 30g

white sugar a spoonful

PROCESS Decoct in an earthenware pot the first two ingredients in 1000ml of cold water over slow fire for half an hour and sift the decoction from the dregs; wash the lotus seed clean and soak them in 300ml of hot water for an hour. Then pour the decoction and the lotus seed with the water into an aluminium pan and stew them on top of slow fire for an hour. Finally add the white sugar to them and stew them for another hour until the lotus seed is well-done.

DIRECTIONS To be taken as snacks. This decoction is especially good for patients suffering from seminal emission manifested as nocturnal emission resulting from hyperactivity of fire due to yin deficiency complicated by mild hypertension.

3) Tortoise Soup for Tonifying the Kidney and Replenishing the Essence of Life (Bushen Yijing Wugui Tang)

INGREDIENTS

desertliving cistanche, Herba Cistanches 60g

Chinese raspberry, Fructus rubi 30g

tortoise, Chinemys reevesii 1000g

PROCESS First soak the desertliving cistanche and the Chinese raspberry in 300ml of thin salt solution for 30 minutes. Then put the meat of the tortoise with its shell, the soaked desertliving cistanche and the Chinese raspberry with the soaking salt solution in a big earthenware pot, and pour in cold water until all of them are inundated. Afterwards, heat them with strong fire. When the water begins to boil, add half a spoonful of fine table salt, and stew them with slow fire for four hours until the shell of the tortoise is disintegrated and the meat is well-done.

DIRECTIONS The soup is to be drunk and the tortoise meat to be eaten. It is to be taken in two days, twice a day, before meals. It is applicable to patients suffering from seminal emission marked by the type of unconsolidation due to kidney deficiency accompanied with the symptom of neurosism.

4) Sweets of Walnut Kernel for Curing Seminal Emission (Gujing Hetao Tang)

INGREDIENTS

dogwood fruit, fructus Corni 250g

schisandra fruit, Fructus Schisandrae 100g

walnut kernel, Semen Juglandis 1000g

crystal sugar 500g

PROCESS Sock the schisandra fruit in cold water in an earthenware pot for half an hour, then decoct is over slow fire until it becomes thick juice. Place the walnut kernel in a big ceramic basin and soak it with the thick juice of schisandra fruit. Half an hour later, mix the dogwood fruit into them and put the crystal sugar on the mixture, then cover the basin and steam with the basin in boiling water for three hours. Steam the sweets every three days, 15 minutes each time.

DIRECTIONS To be taken with warm boiled water after chewed carefully, 3 times a day, 10g each time. This recipe can regulate and bring down blood pressure, so it is applicable to both the old and the middle-aged who suffer from nocturnal emission and neurosism accompanied with hypertension due to kidney deficiency.

Section 18

Prostatic Hyperplasia

This disease is manifested mainly as frequent urination, more frequent at night, which affects sleep, afterwards the urine stream can be seen having got narrower, the range having got shorter and the time for urination having lasted longer, and distending pain in the lower abdomen. It falls in TCM into the category of "long bi"(retention of urine)

1. **Common Types of Syndromes**

1) Deficiency-cold of the Lower-jiao Manifested as frequent urination, bradyuria, dripping urination, cold extremities, soreness of the loins and legs, pale tongue, deep and thready pulse.

2) Stagnation of Damp-heat Manifested as difficulty in urination, dripping urination, unbearable difficulty and pain in micturition, distending pain in the abdomen, yellow and greasy fur, slippery and rapid pulse.

2. **Composite Medicated Diet**

1) Kidneys Stewed with Eucommia Bark (Duzhong Yaohua)

INGREDIENTS

sheep kidney (or pork kidney) 2

eucommia bark , Cortex Eucommiae 15g

ginger, Rhizoma Zingiberis Recens right amount

green Chinese onion, Bulbus Allii Fistulosi right amount

table salt right amount

PROCESS Cut the kidneys open, get rid of the membrane; then stew them together with all the other ingredients until the kidneys are done.

DIRECTIONS The kidneys are to be eaten. Applicable to patients suffering from prostatic hyperplasia of deficiency cold of the lower-jiao.

2) Decoction of Aniseed and Chinese Green Onion (Huxiang Congbai Jian)

aniseed, Fructus Foeniculi 5g

Chinese green onin, Bulbus Allii Fistulosi 4

PROCESS AND DIRECTIONS Pound them together and decoct them for oral administration. To be taken in three separate doses. Applicable to patients suffering from prostatic hyperplasia of deficiency-cold of lower-jiao.

3) Mung Bean Gruel (Qingxiaodou Zhou)

INGREDIENTS

mung bean, Semen Phaseoli Radiati 80g

wheat, Fructus Tritici 50g

ricepaper pith, Medulla Tetrapanacis 10g

PROCESS　Decoct the last ingredient in water and remove the dregs, and then make gruel with the decoction and the first two ingredients.

DIRECTIONS　To be taken as breakfast. Applicable to patients suffering from prostatic hyperplasia of stagnation of damp-heat.

Section 19

Urolithiasis

Urolithiasis is the general term for calculi at the different parts of the urinary system, and it is one of the major disorder in this system. The cause of urolithiasis is very complicated, and it is considered to be closely related to the environmental factors, affections of the whole body and the urinary system. The clinical characteristics of this disease are lumbago, hematuria dysuria and urodynia. This affection belongs to the category of "urination disturbance" in the lore of traditional Chinese medicine. The mechanism of the disease is chiefly due to the accumulation of damp-heat in the lower burner, thus giving rise to an unfavourable gasification of the urinary bladder. Though the diseased sites are at the urinary bladder and the kidney, they are closely related to the liver and the spleen.

The basic principle for treatment is: In case of excess, sedative method is used; in case of deficiency, tonifying method is used.

Medicated diet has a certain curative effect on both alleviating the symptoms and helping remove the calculi.

1. Common Type of Syndromes

Stagnation of Damp-heat　Manifested as gripping pain in the waist and abdomen, which affects the lower abdomen, or radiates toward perineum, frequent micturition, urgent urination, urodynia, difficult prolonged scanty urination, blood in the urine, sometimes there are stones in the urine, red tongue with thick yellow and greasy fur, wiry and rapid pulse or slippery and rapid pulse.

2. **Composite Medicated Diet**

1)Decoction of Lysimachia and Chicken's Gizzard (Jinqiancao Jizhin Tang)

INGREDIENTS

dried lysimachia, Herba Lysimachiae 50g

chickens gizzard 2

PROCESS Place the two ingredients in a small earthenware pot, pour cold water into it until they are inundated; then stew them over soft fire for an hour.

DIRECTIONS To be taken twice a day, 300ml of the soup and one chicken's gizzard each time. The soup is to be drunk and the gizzard is to be taken along with bread or rice after cut into slices and dipped in soy sauce, 15 to 30 days making up one course of treatment. This decoction can dissolve stones.

2)Decoction of Corn Stigma and Cogongrass Rhizome (Yumixu Baimaogen Tang)

INGREDIENTS

corn stigma, Stigma Maydis 30g

cogongrass rhizome, Rhizoma Imperatae 30g

Chinese-date, Fructus Ziziphi Jujubae 8

PROCESS Put all the three ingredients in a small aluminium pan with 1500 ml of cold water and cook them over soft fire for 30 to 40 minutes.

DIRECTIONS To be taken twice a day 500ml each time. The decoction is to be drunk and the dates to be eaten, one month making up one course of treatment. This recipe can lead up to the best result when taken by patients suffering from incipient ureteral calculus or vesical calculus marked by dark urine, red blood cells in urine proved by uroscopy accompanied with hypertension.

3)Decoction of Stalk Pith of Sunflower (Xiangrikui Jingxin Tang)

INGREDIENTS

stalk pith of fresh sunflower, Medulla Hellianthi annui 50g

(or 20g of that of dried sunflower)

talc, Talcum 10g

honey, Mel 1 spoonful

PROCESS Decoct in 1000 ml of cold water the first two ingredients in an earthenware pot; when the liquid is boiled down to 300 ml, sift the decoction from the dregs and mix honey into it.

DIRECTIONS To be taken as a drink every day. This recipe can treat stranguria and is good for diuresis, and what is more, it has no side effect. It can also relieve summer-heat when drunk in summer.

4) Drink of Climbing Fern Spore and Tea (Haijinsha Cha)

INGREDIENTS

climbing fern spore, Spora Lygodii 15g

green tea (the oldest the best), Folium Camelliae Viride 2g

PROCESS Infuse both of them in boiling water in a glass.

DIRECTIONS Take one glass first before meals after getting up every morning, then take it any time as you please. Two months make up one course of treatment.

All the recipes stated above are appicable to the type of stagnation of damp-heat; those who suffer from stone of urinary system can select any of them to eat.

Section 20

Diabetes

Diabetes is a frequently seen disorder of endocrinal metabolism. Its fundamental pathologic and physiologic base is the absolute or relative insufficiency of insulin, thus giving rise to disturbance of sugar metabolism, later inducing successive disturbance of metabolism of protein, fat, vitamin, water and electrolyte. The clinical characteristics of the disease are: Polydipsia, polyphagia but getting thinner, polyuria or turbid urine.

In TCM, it belongs to the categories of consumption and thirst, the special feature of the mechanism of disease is that deficiency of yin is the root cause and dry heat is the symptom. The affection is at the organs of lung, stomach and kidney. On basis of the clinical characteristics and the mechanism of disease, recuperation by proper diet plays a very important role in relieving the above symptoms of the patients. Therefore, dietetic Chinese drugs and medicated diet are comparatively desirable aids in treating this disease.

1. **Common Types of Syndromes**

1)Scorching action of stomach—fire and impairment of body fluid due to dryness of the lung Marked by extreme thirst and excessive drinking, dry mouth and tongue, normal discharge of excrement with frequent urine, red margin and tip of the tongue with thin, yellow coating and rapid pulse.

2)Excessiveness of stomach—fire and insufficiency of yin fluid Marked by extreme thirst and excessive drinking, polyorexia, constipation, yellow and dry coating on the tongue and smooth and rapid pulse.

3)Deficiency and exhaustion of vital essence and energy and unconsolidation of the kidney—qi Marked by polyuria, turbid urine, dizziness and waist—soreness, dry mouth and red tongue, deep and thready pulse.

2. **Composite of Medicated Diet**

1)Drink of Five Juices(Wu Zhi Yin Fang)

INGREDIENTS

pear juice, Malum Piri

water chestnut juice, Bulbus Heleocharis Tuberosae

juice of fresh reed rhizome, Rhizoma Phragmitis Recens

juice of lilyturf root, Radix Ophiopogonis

lotus root juice, Rhizoma Nelumbinis

PROCESS Mix thoroughly the five kinds of juices, of pear, water chestnut , fresh reed rhizome, lilyturf root and lotus root.

DIRECTIONS Take it cool. The amount of each juice is decided spontaneously. Applicable to patient suffering from diabetes of the types of scorching action of stomach—fire and impairment of body due to dryness of the lung, and excessiveness of the stomach—fire and insufficiency of yin fluid.

2)Gruel of Rehmannia Root(Shengdihuang Zhou)

INGREDIENTS

juice of rehmannia root, Radix Rehmanniae 150 ml

long—stored millet, Semen Setariae Italicae

PROCESS Add 150ml of rehmannia root juice into the gruel made from long—stored millet.

DIRECTIONS Stir and mix it thoroughly for eating. Applicable to patient suffering from diabetes of the types of scorching action of stomch—fire and impairment of body due to dryness of the lung, and excessiveness of stomach—fire and insufficiency of yin fluid.

3)Soup of Pork Skin(Zhufu Tang)

INGREDIENTS

pork skin 500g

rice flour 250g

PROCESS Decoct 500g of pork skin and 250g of rice flour in water until it smells fragrant, stir and mix it thoroughly.

DIRECTIONS Take it warm in six times.

4)Pudding of Hempseed and Chestnut Powder(Maren Lizi Gao)

INGREDIENTS

hempseed, Fructus Cannabis

sesame seed, Semen Sesami

chestnut powder, Pulvis Castaneae

corn flour

PROCESS Steam corn flour mixed with hempseeds , sesame seeds and chestnut powder into puddings for eating.

5)Eggs Stewed with Schisandra Fruit(Wuweizi Dun Dan)

INGREDIENTS

eggs(hen's or pigeon's)

schisandra fruit, Fructus Schisandrae

PROCESS Stew eggs together with schisandra fruit for eating.

The three recipes cited above can be used to treat the type of deficiency and exhaustion of the vital essence and energy due to unconsolidation of the lower—jiao.

Section 21

Hyperlipemia

Hyperlipemia(HL)is a kind of disease in which one or more kinds of plasma lipids extend their normal limit. In clinical practice, HL is classified into two types: the primary and the secondary types. The secondary type is caused by abnormal metabolism of plasma lipids and lipoprotein(LP) in diabetes, diseases of the liver, pancrea, and gallbladder etc. This syndrome usually has symptoms such as drowsy heaviness in the head, stuffiness in the chest and abdomen, and so on. Some patients may have no apparent symptoms and do not suffer much.

In TCM, HL belongs to the categories of "phlegm—damp", "turbid blockage", "blood stasis" etc., and is considered to be related to the spleen, liver and kidney. Its general mechanisms are yin deficiency of the liver and kidney, the stasis of liver qi and falling to send up essential substances in the physiologic functions of the spleen.

When treating HL, one should consider both the principal and secondary aspects of the disease. In the aspect of treating the principal, tonifying the kidney, harmonizing the liver and strengthening the spleen are required; In the aspect of treating the secondary, promoting digestion and relieving stasis, eliminating phlegm and excreting damp, clearing heat and dissolving stagnated blood should be focused.

Dietetic Chinese drugs and recipes of composite medicated diet cited here are applicable not only to those who have apparent clinical symptoms of hyperlipemia, but also to those who have subclinical symptoms with really high blood—lipid level if examined.

1. **Common Type of Syndromes**

1) Stagnation phlegm—turbidity Manifested as drowsy heaviness in head, sensation of stuffiness in the chest and abdomen, or nausea, or a full figure with a short breath, heaviness sensation in the body, numbness and heaviness of the limbs, white greasy or moist coating on the tongue, and taut and slippery pulse.

2) Yin deficiency in the liver and kidney Manifested as dizziness and headache, dry eyes and blurred , amnesia, tinnitus, palpitation, insomnia, soreness of the waist, numbness of the limbs, dry mouth, a little reddish tongue, thin or rapid pulse.

3) Stasis of the liver Qi Manifested as dizziness or headache, distension and pain in the right costal region (or whole costal region) and the gastric cavity, apparently aggravated by emotional fluctuation; mental irritability at ordinary time; or dullness and depression, red tongue with thin—white or thin—yellow fur, taut pulse.

2. **Composite of Medicated Diet**

1) Gruel of Fleece—flower Root (Heshouwu Zhou)

INGREDIENTS

fleece—flower root, Radix Polygoni Mulitflori (powdered)

polished round—grained rice, Semen Oryzae Sativae 50g

Chinese—date, Fructus Ziziphi Jujubae 2

white sugar right amount

PROCESS Wash fleece—flower root clean and dry it the sun; then grind it into fine powder. Choose 50g of first—class polished round—grained rice, two Chinese—dates, right amount of white sugar and put them all into an earthenware pot; add 500ml of water and cook them together to make thin gruel. Then, put the powdered fleece—flower root (20 to 30g at a time); stir it gently to mix it thoroughly; go on cooking it over a slow fire until it has boiled several times. Stop cooking when the gruel is thick and sticky. Cover the pot tight for five minutes.

DIRECTIONS Take it warm at one draught, twice a day, at breakfast and at supper. The gruel can exert a tonic effect on the heart, lower blood lipid and blood pressure. Do not use an ironware to cook the gruel.

2) Gruel of Lotus Leaf (Heye Zhou)

INGREDIENTS

polished round—grained rice, Semen Oryzae Sativae 50g

crystal sugar right amount

fresh lotus leaf, Folium Nelumbinis1

PROCESS Cut one fresh lotus leaf into thin slices and decoct it in water so as to get about 150ml of thick extract; get rid of the dregs from the extract and put in 50g of polished round—grained rice, right amount of crystal sugar and 400ml of water, getting them cooked together to make mediumthick gruel.

DIRECTIONS Take the gruel warm, twice a day. It is especially fit to be taken in summer. Having a delicate fragrance, this kind of gruel is particularly peptizing, a fit to be taken over a long period of time by the aged who suffer from hypertension and hyperlipemia.

Section 22

Simple Obesity

Simple obesity refers to non—pathologic adiposity. The body weight of such patients is 20% heavier than the body weight based on the criteria recommended by WHO. The normal way of calculation is: body—height(cm)—100/105=the standard body weight of men/women. The major pathologic change is the increase of the number or the enlargement of the volume of adipose tissues.

According to the TCM lore, the basic mechanism of this affection is deficiency of Qi, and phlegm—turbidity is the product of pathology. Deficiency of Qi is closely related very much to the spleen and kidney. Weakness or disorders of spleen and kidney is the pathologic base of obesity.

1. **Common Type of Syndromes**

The common syndrome is stagnation of phlegm—dampness with insufficiency of the spleen and qi, manifested as obesity, sluggishness of heavy limbs, impeded movement; sometimes marked by dizziness, shortness of breath, fullness and choking sensation in the chest and stomach, enlarged tongue with white and greasy, or yellow and white coating, slippery or deep and relaxed pulse.

2. **Composite of Medicated Diet**

Lotus Leaf and Hawthorn Fruit Drink(Heye Shanzha Yin)

INGREDIENTS

lotus leaf, Folium Nelumbinis 9g

hawthorn fruit, Fructus Crataegi(Powdered) 9g

PROCESS Decoct 9g of lotus leaf and 9g burnt hawthorn fruit in water for a while and take it as a drink. To treat simple obesity, it is advisable to take such a drink frequently.

Section 23

Viral Hepatitis

This disease has two major types: icteric and non—icteric. Icterohepatitis belongs to the category of "huangdan"(jaundice) in traditional Chinese medicine, marked by icteric sclera and skin, and yellow—coloured urine; while nonicteric hepatitis the categories of "xie tong"(hypochrondriac Pain),"yu zheng"(disturbance of the liver — qi) marked by nausea, hypochrondriac pain, distension and fullness in the abdomen and lassitude.

Medicated dietetic treatment is an auxiliary aid of great importance to the treatment of the disease, which plays a role not ignorable in relieving the patient's symptoms, and recuperating the health of the organisms.

1. **Common Types of syndromes**

1) Biliation due to damp—heat accumulating in the liver and gallbladder

Marked by icteric sclera and skin, and yellow—coloured urine, accompanied with fever, irritability, nausea and vomiting, loss of appetite, yellowish and greasy fur on the tongue, and taut and rapid pulse.

2) Accumulation of excessive damp—heat in the interior due to incoordination between the spleen and the stomach   Marked by nausea, hypochondriac pain, distension and fullness in the abdomen, lassitude, accompanied with loss of appetite, irritability, white and greasy or yellowish and greasy fur on the tongue, and slippery and rapid pulse.

3) Stagnation of qi and blood resulting from incoordinaiton between the liver and the spleen   Marked by wandering or stationary distending pain or piercing pain in the hypochondrium, dim complexion, loss of appetite, distension in the abdomen, belching or hepatosplenomegaly, dim and pale tongue or with ecchymoses, thin fur on the tongue, and taut and uneven pulse.

2. **Composite Recipes of Medicated Diet**

1) Gruel with Oriental Wormwood (Yinchen Zhou)

INGREDIENTS

oriental wormwood, Herba Artemisiae Capillaris 30 to 45g

polished round—grained rice, Semen Oryzae Sativae 100g

white sugar a bit

PROCESS   Have some oriental wormwood washed clean and use 30 to 45g at a time; add 200 ml of water and decoct it until 100 ml of water is left. Remove the dregs to get the extract; put in 100g of polished round — grained rice, add 600ml of water and cook until the rice is well—done and the extract becomes thick. Add a bit of white sugar and go on cooking for a while until it has boiled for a little while.

DIRECTIONS   Take it 2 or 3 times a day, with 7 to 10 days as a course of treatment. It can be applied to acute icterohepatitis marked by the type of bile oozing from the gallbladder due to damp—heat accumulating in the liver and gallbladder.

2)Recipe of Giant Knotweed Rhizome and Honey (Huzhang Mi)

INGREDIENTS

giant knotweed rhizome, Rhizoma Polygoni Cuspitati 500g

schisandra fruit, Fructus Schisandrae 250g

honey, Mel 1000g

PROCESS Wash the giant knotweed rhizome and schisandra fruit clean, put them in an earthenware pot and add water (to the point that the two drugs can be submerged) and soak them for half an hour. Heat them over a moderate fire until the water boils. Then, change to a low fire and go on decocting for about half an hour until 500ml of medicinal extract is left; filter it to get the extract. Add 1000ml of water and heat it to get extract of about 500 ml; remove the dregs and put all the extract obtained and the honey into a big earthenware pot which is to be heated over a low fire. Let the decoction boil for 5 minutes, take the pot away from the fire to let it cool. Pour the decoction in a bottle and cover it tight.

DIRECTIONS Take a spoonful at a fime after meals, three times a day after infusing it with boiling water, with two months as a course of treatment.

3) Decoction of Oriental Wormwood, Germinated Barley and Jujube (Yinchen Maiya Hongzao Tang)

INGREDIENTS

oriental wormwood, Herba Artemisiae Capillaris 15g

germinated barley, Fructus Hordei Germinatus 20g

jujube, Fructus Ziziphi Jujubae 10

white sugar a bit

PROCESS Put the oriental wormwood, germinated barley and jujubes in a small aluminium pan, add 1000ml of cold water to stew the drugs slowly over a low fire for about half an hour; put in a half spoonful of white sugar and take it away from the fire.

DIRECTIONS Take less than half a bowlful at a time, twice a day. Drink the decoction, eat the jujubes and discard the dregs.

The above composite recipes are applicable to both the type of incoordination between the liver and the stomach caused by damp—heat accumulating in the interior, and the type of stagnancy of qi and blood in acute and chronic hepatitis. It can be used as an auxiliary treatment for chronic hepatitis patients.

Section 24

Pulmonary Tuberculosis

It is also termed "fei lao" or "lao zhai" (consumptive disease) in traditional Chinese medicine, marked by cough, hemoptysis, tidal fever, night sweat and gradual emaciation.

1. **Common Types of Syndromes**

1) Deficiency of the lung—yin Marked by dry cough with little phlegm, or sputum mixed with blood, tidal fever, night sweat, flushing of zygomatic region, dry pharynx and mouth, reddened tongue, and thready and rapid pulse.

2) Insufficiency of the lung—qi and the spleen—qi Marked by short breath, cough with sputum, tightness of the chest, loss of appetite, listlessness, low and weak voice, pale complexion, aversion to cold, white and greasy fur on the tongue, and thready and feeble pulse.

3) Insufficiency of both the lung—qi and the lung—yin Marked by cough with little sputum, or blood tinged sputum, short breath and listlessness, flushing of zygomatic region and pale complexion, spontaneous and night sweat, dry pharynx and mouth, loss of appetite, reddened tongue with white or exfoliative fur, and thready, rapid and feeble pulse.

2. **Composite Recipes of Medicated Diet**

1) Recipe of Sichuan Fritillary Bulb, Fragrant Solomonseal Rhizome and Crystal Sugar (Chuanbei Yuzhu Bingtang Fang)

INGREDIENTS

Sichuan fritillary bulb, Bulbus Fritillariae Cirrhosae
(pounded into pieces) 6 to 9g
fragrant solomonseal rhizone, Rhizoma Polygonati Odorati 15g
crystal sugar 25g

PROCESS Stew the ingredients in just the right amount of water for oral administration.

DIRECTIONS Take it twice a day, for 15 to 20 days successively.

2) Decoction of Chinese Caterpillar Fungus and Tremella (chongcao Yiner Tang)

INGREDIENTS

Chinese caterpillar fungus, Cordyceps 10g

tremella, Tremella 15g

crystal (or white) sugar 30g

PROCESS Have the Chinese caterpillar fungus washed clean and wrapped up; put it into a small earthenware pot together with the tremella and crystal sugar. Stew it slowly over a low fire for 2 to 3 hours; take it away from the fire and remove the packet of Chinese caterpillar fungus (Wash the gauze clean and keep it for use next time).

DIRECTIONS Take a small bowlful at a time, twice a day, once in the morning on an empty stomach and once in the evening before going to bed; gargle after eating it.

The two recipes listed above are applicable to cases with the type of deficiency of the lung—yin.

3) Soup of Dangshen, Lily Bulb and Pork Lung (Shen He Zhufei Tang)

INGREDIENTS

dangshen, Radix Codonopsis pilosulae 15g

lily bulb, Bulbus Lilii 30g

pork lung 250g

PROCESS Stew the above ingredients in just the right amount of water over a low fire, season them after well done.

DIRECTIONS Drink the soup and eat the pork lung. Take it twice in a day, for 15 to 20 days successively.

4) Gruel of Hyacinth Bletilla, Polished Round—grained Rice and Garlic (Baiji Mi Suan Zhou)

INGREDIENTS

garlic with purplish skins, Bulbus Allii 30g

polished round—grained rice, Semen Oryzae Sativae 60g

powder of hyacinth bletilla, Rhizoma Bletillae 5g

PROCESS Cook the rice and the powder of hyacinth bletilla in water until they are well done; then , put in the prepared garlic (remove the skins, boil it in boiling water for a minute, and then take it out) and cook it in the gruel.

DIRECTIONS　Take this kind of gruel frequently in the morning and in the evening, and that often.

The two recipes listed above are all applicable to cases with the type of insufficiency of the lung—qi and the spleen—qi.

5) Soup of Radish and Mutton (Luobo Yangrou Tang)

INGREDIENTS

mutton (from legs of a sheep or a goat) 1000g

white radish, Napus 500g

carrot, Radix Dauci Carotae 60g

fresh ginger, Rhizoma Zingiberis Recens 3 slices

peel of 2 tangerines, Pericarpium Citri Reticulatae

PROCESS　Have the white radish , carrot, mutton washed clean and cut into cubes, put three spoonfuls of vegetable oil into a pan that is heated over a brisk fire; first, put in the ginger and fry it quickly after the oil becomes hot, then, put in the mutton immediately, stirfry it for five minutes, add three spoonfuls of rice (or millet) wine, fry it until it gives off fragrance, add half a bowlful of cold water, go on heating so as to let it boil for ten minutes, Ladle it out. Put the mutton, carrot and dried tangerine peel into a big earthenware pot, add cold water to submerge all the ingredients; after it has boiled over a moderate fire, add a spoonful of rice (or millet) wine, one and a half spoonfuls of refined salt; change to cooking it over a low fire for half an hour, add the white radish. Go on cooking it over a low fire for an hour; when the mutton, radish are thoroughly done, stop cooking.

DIRECTIONS　Discard the tangerine peel, take the rest with bread (or cooked rice). It is most suitable for eating in severe winter.

6) Soup of Soft—shelled Turtle Flesh and Stemona Root (Bierou Baibu Tang)

INGREDIENTS

soft—shelled turtle flesh, Trionyx Sinensis 250g

stemona roots , Radix Stemonae 15g

wolfberry bark, Cortex Lycii Radicis 15g

dried root of rehmannia, Radix Rehmanniae 20g

astragalus root, Radix Astragali seu Hedysari 15g

PROCESS Decoct the above ingredients in water and take it after removing the medicinal dregs.

DIRECTIONS Take a dose a day, for 7 to 10 days suceesively.

The two recipes listed above applicable to cases with the type of insufficiency of the lung—qi and the lung—yin.

Section 25

Neurosism

Neurosism is a morbid condition resulting from the temporal functional disorder of cerebral certex caused by psychic factors. It is marked mainly by insomnia and dreamful sleep, dizziness and feeling of fullness in the head, palpitation, hypomnesis, alopecia, and spermatorrhea.

It belongs to the categories of "jingji"(palpitation due to fright)。"bumei" (insomnia), "jian wang" (amnesia), "xuanyun" (dizziness), "toutong" (headache), "xusun"(comsumptive disease) and so on, in the science of traditional Chinese medicine. Medicated diet therapy is beneficial both to relieving the symptoms and to the recovery of organism.

1. Common Types of Syndromes

1) Flame upward of liver—fire and burn of heart—yin Palpitation, dysphoria, irritability accompanied with insomnia and excessive dreaming, tinnitus and dizziness, flushed face, dark urine, red tongue with little fur, and wiry rapid pulse.

2) Deficiency of qi, blood, heart and spleen Palpitation and insomnia, dreaminess and propensity to wake, timidness and aptness to the frightened, accompanied with dizziness and amnesia, anorexia, lassitude of the mind and body, pale tongue with teeth prints at its borders, and deep, thready and weak pulse.

3) Hyperactivity of fire due to yin deficiency and disharmony between the heart and the kidney Manifested as palpitation, insomnia due to vexation, accompanied with propensity to be frightened while sleeping or dreaming, sponta-

neous sweating at night, lassitude in the loins and legs, seminal emission, red tongue, and thready and rapid pulse.

2. Composite Recipes of Medicated Diet

1) Decoction with Dried Longan Aril and Arborvitae Seeds (Guiyuan Baiziren Tang)

INGREDIENTS

longan aril, Arillus Longan 10g

arborvitae seed, Semen Biotae 10g

PROCESS Put 10g of dried longan aril and 10g of arborvitae seeds together into a small aluminium pan, add 500ml of cold water and half a spoonful of white sugar, cook them together on a slow fire for 20 to 30 minutes until about 200 ml of extract is left, then take the pan away from the fire, remove the residues of the arborvitae seeds

DIRECTIONS Take it twice a day.

It is applicable to deficiency of qi, blood, heart and spleen.

2) Soft Extract for Calming the Liver, Invigorating the Spleen and Tranquilizing the Mind (Pinggan Yipi Anshen Gao)

INGREDIENTS

longan aril, Arillus Longan 1000g

(or 250g of dried longan aril)

Chinese-date, Fructus Ziziphi Jujubae 500g

prunella spike, Spica Prunellae 200g

spiny jujube seed, Semen Ziziphi Spinosae 100g

honey, Mel 1000g

crystal sugar 250g

PROCESS Put the Chinese-dates, prunella spike and spiny jujube seeds into a big earthenware pot and soak them in cold water for half an hour and then, heat it over a medium fire. When the water boils, decoct it over a slow fire for an hour until 1000ml or so of extract is left; filter it to get the first extract; add 1500ml of cold water into the pot and heat it again until 700 ml of medicinal fluid is left; filter it to get the second extract and remove the residues. Put all the extract, the dried longan aril, honey and crystal sugar into the big earthenware pot and heat it over a slow fire for about an hour. Cool it to have soft syrupy extract, and then, put it into a bottle and cover it tight.

DIRECTIONS Take it after its infusion with boiling water, twice a day, 10 to 15g at a time. As for the longan aril, swallow it after chewing it. It is very effective for those who suffer from the flaring of liver—fire marked by irritability accompanied with high blood pressure if they take this kind of soft extract frequently over a long period of time.

It is applicable to the type of syndrome in which liver—flares up and burns the heart—yin.

3) Decoction with Dragon's Bone, Oyster Shell and Lotus Seed (Longgu Muli Lianzi Tang)

INGREDIENTS

dragon's bone, Os Draconis Fossilia Ossis Mastodi 10g

oyster shell, Concha Ostreae 15g

rhizome of wind—weed, Rhizoma Anemarrhenae 3g

lotus seed, Semen Nelumbinis 30g

PROCESS Decoct the dragon's bone and oyster shell first, then put in the rhizome of wind—weed, lotus seeds and white sugar to make decoction for drinking. It exerts a remarkable effect upon those suffering from insomnia, night sweat, dysphoria with smothery sensation and is applicable to the type of hyperactivity of fire due to yin deficiency with break—down of the normal physiological coordination between the heart and the kidney.

4) Honey with Sesame Seed and Three Kinds of Kernels (San Ren Zhima Mi)

INGREDIENTS

spiny jujube seed, Semen Ziziphi Spinosae 60g

arborvitae seed, Semen Biotae 60g

hemp seeds, Fructus Cannabis 30g

black seasame seed, Semen Sesami Nigrum 500g

honey, Mel 500g

PROCESS First, decoct the arborvitae seeds, hemp seeds and spiny jujube seeds; put the first and the second extract obtained separately and honey into an earthenware pot to be heated over a small fire. When it boils, put in the roasted black sesame seeds, stir it continuously with a chopstick for a quarter of an hour, then, remove the pot from the fire. Put the content into a bottle after it cools.

DIRECTIONS Take it twice a day, 10g at a time, after infusing it with boiling water or take it with cooked rice (or millet) water. As for the sesame seeds, swallow it after is chewing. This recipe is especially fit for the aged patients who suffer from neurosism.

Section 26

Cerebrovascular Diseases

Diseases including cerebral hemorrhage, cerebral thrombosis, cerebral embolism, subarachnoid hemorrhage, hypertensive cerephalopathy and so on, all belong to the category of "zhong—feng" (apoplexy) in TCM.

The clinical characteristics of this disease are sudden attacks, facial hemiparalysis, retarded speech or hemiplegia in the mild type; sudden fall and coma in the severe case.

1. **Common Types of Syndromes**

1) Accumulation in the interior of the phlegm and heat Manifested as regaining consciousness after a fainting spell, uttering a sigh and opening the mouth, laryngeal rale, retarded speech , stiff tongue with greasy fur and deep, slippery and forceful pulse.

2) Blazing of the liver—fire M marked by uttering a sigh and opening the mouth after a fainting spell, raucous breathing, restlessness, accompanied with feeling of distension in the head, tinnitus, parietal headache, red margin of the tongue, and wiry and rapid pulse.

3) Vital—qi tending to break Manifested as closing eyes and opening the mouth, hoarseness and raucous breathing, shortened tongue and darkish complexion, spontaneous perspiration, limbs with coldness extending up to the elbows and knees, involuntary passage of urine and feces, pale tongue, and deep, thready and weak pulse.

4) Deficiency of the kidney and blockade of the channels and collaterals

Marked by shortened tongue with difficulty on speaking, flaccidity of the feet with difficulty in walking, hemiplegia, reddish tongue, thready and weak pulse.

2. Composite Recipes of Medicated Diet

1)Gruel of Bamboo Juice(Zhuli Zhou)

INGREDIENTS

juice of henon bamboo, succus Bambosae

millet, Semen setariae Italicae

PROCESS Get henon bamboo juice (excreted from the baked bamboo stem) and millet, each equal in portion; first, make gruel with the millet, and when it is done, put in the bamboo juice.

DIRECTIONSS tir and mix it thoroughly for taking the gruel warm, twice a day. it is especially fit to be taken in summer, and applicable to the type of the accumulation in the interior of phlegm and heat of "zhong feng". It can have a curative effect after taking it a long period of time.

2)Decoction of Schisandra Fruit(Wuweizi Tang)

INGREDIENTS

schisandra fruit, fructus Schisandrae 10g

purple perilla leaves, Folium Perillae 18g

ginseng, Radix Ginseng 12g

granulated sugar 100g

PROCESS Get 10g of schisandra fruit, 18g of purple perilla leaves, 12g of ginseng and 100g of granulated sugar. Decoct the first three drugs in 3000ml of water until 1500ml is left; remove the dregs and let it settle; and add in the granulated sugar.

DIRECTIONS It can be taken as much as one likes. A good preventive effect on the syndrome of feeble vital—qi tending to break, so patients who suffer from this syndrome may take it. It can have a curative effect after a long period of time.

3)Powder of Pig's Bile and Green Gram(Zhudan Ludou Fen)

INGREDIENTS

pig's bile, Succus Fellis Suillum 120g

flour of green gram, Semen Phaseoli Radiati 80g

PROCESS

Mix 80g of green gram flour thoroughly with 120g of pig's bile and dry it by airing, then, grind it into fine powder.

DIRECTIONS

Take 6g at a time, twice a day. It is applicable to the type of blazing of liver—fire.

4) Gruel of Rehmannia Root (Dihuang Zhou)

INGREDIENTS

juice of rehmannia root, Succus Radicis Rehmanniae 100ml

polished round—grained rice, Semen oryzae Sativae

PROCESS Get 100ml of the juice of rehmannia roots ready for use; first, make gruel with polished round—grained rice and when it is done, put in the juice of rehmannia root.

DIRECTIONS Stir and mix thoroughly before eating. It is applicable to the type of deficiency of the kidney and blockade of the channels and collaterals.

Section 27

Anemia

Anemia, a collective name for iron-deficiency anemia, macrocytic anemia, hemolytic anemia, aplastic anemia and other secondary anemia, is characterized by pale or sallow and lusterless complexion, pale lips and finger—nails, sleepiness, lassitude, shortness of breath, dizziness, palpitation due to exertion, emaciation and bleeding. It belongs in TCM to "xue xu" (blood deficiency), "xu lao" (consumptive disease) and "xu huang" (sallow complexion of insufficiency type).

1. Common Types of Syndromes

1) Deficiency of the Heart, Spleen, Qi and Blood In addition to the characteristics stated above, it is also marked by little taste for food, low voice, deficient and feeble pulse; also it may be manifested as nose—bleeding, bleeding from the gums, or dermorrhagia; or in the case of women, scanty and pale menstruation, or amenorrhea if it is a severe case.

2) Deficiency of the Liver—yin, Kidney—yin, Essence and Blood Manifested as dizziness, conjunctival congestion, tinnitus, lassitude in the loins and legs, seminal emission and night sweat, flushing of zygomatic region and tidal fever, feverish sensation in the palms and soles, red tongue, thready and rapid

pulse.

3)Deficiency of both the Blood and Qi with Insufficiency of the Spleen—yang and Kidney—yang Besides the characteristics of anemia, it is marked by aversion to cold, coldness of extremities, lassitude, disinclination to speak, perspiration, loose stools, pale tongue with white fur, deep and thready pulse.

2. **Composite Medicated Diet**

1)Pills of Soybean and Green Copperas(Huangdou Zaofan Wan)

INGREDIENTS

parched soybean, Semen Glycinis 60g

calcined green copperas, Ferrosi Sulfas Crudus 30g

Chinese—date, Fructus Ziziphi Jujubae

PROCESS Grind the first two ingredients into fine powder; then decoct Chinese—dates in water; finally make pills with the powder and the decoction.

DIRECTIONS To be taken twice a day, 6g each time. Green copperas contains ferrous sulfate, so this recipe can be used to treat iron—deficiency anemia, and is applicable to the type of deficiency of the heart, spleen, qi and blood.

2)Soup of Asia Bell, Chinese Angelica Root and Pigeon Meat(Shen Gui Gerou Tang)

INGREDIENTS

pigeon, Columba Livia Domestica 1

Asia bell, Radix Codonopsis Pilosulae 25g

Chinese angelica root, Radix Angelicae Sinensis 12g

PROCESS Stew all the ingredients in water.

DIRECTIONS The soup is to be taken orally for treating anemia of the type of deficiency of both the blood and qi with insufficiency of the spleen—yang and kidney—yang.

3)Thick Soup of Cherry and Longan Aril(Yingtao Long yan Geng)

INGREDIENTS

longan aril, Arillus Longan 10g, or fresh longan aril 15g

wolfberry fruit, Fructus Lycii 10g

fresh cherry, Fructus Pseudocerasi 30g

white sugar

PROCESS First, decoct the first two ingredients together in a right amount of water. After they have expanded to the full extent, put in the cherry and continue to decoct them until they are brought to the boil; then season them with white sugar.

DIRECTIONS To be taken orally. Every 100g of cherry contains 5. 9mg of iron, so this recipe is applicable to iron-deficiency anemia. Those who suffer from anemia of the type of deficiency of the liver—yin, kidney—yin, essence and blood can take it.

Section 28

Thrombopenic Purpura

This disease is a trouble mainly manifested as bleeding In TCM, dermorrhagia due to this disease belongs to "fa ban"(purpura), "hong zhen"(petechial hemorrhage), "ji nu"(hematohidrosis); while visceral hemorrhage belongs to "xue zheng"(blood troubles). Medicated diet has a certain curative effect on this disease.

1. **Common Types of Syndromes**

1) Excessive Accumulation of Toxic Heat Manifested as purple ecchymoses, or epistaxis, bleeding from the gums, hematuria, hematochezia, irritability, red tongue with yellow fur, wiry and rapid pulse.

2) Interior Heat due to Yin Deficiency Marked by more purple ecchymoses, profuse bleeding with bright red blood, accompanied with tidal fever, vexation, feverish sensation in the palms and soles, red tongue with dry fur, thready and rapid pulse.

3) Failure of Qi to Keep the Blood Flowing within the Vessels Manifested as repeated bleeding, ecchymoses on the whole body, accompanied with epistaxis, bleeding from the gums, dizziness, pale complexion, lusterless lips and finger nails, mental and bodily tiredness, palpitation, shortness of breath due to exertion, pale tongue, wiry, thready and weak pulse.

2. **Composite Medicated Diet**

1) Decoction of Pigskin and Cogongrass (Zhupi Maogen Jian)

INGREDIENTS

cogongrass rhizome, Rhizoma Imperatae 60g

pigskin, Corium Suis 500g

crystal sugar right amount

PROCESS Deccoct the cogongrass rhizome (wrapped in cloth) in water. After getting rid of the hair of the pigskin and washing it clean, stew it with the decoction. When they become thick and sticky, mix it with crystal sugar.

DIRECTIONS To be taken 4 to 5 times, once a day and several doses in succession. It is applicable to patients suffering from the type of excessive accumulation of toxic heat.

2) Decoction of Tree Peony Bark, Fresh — Water Turtle Shell and Dried Rehmannia Root (Danpi Biejia Shengdi Tang)

INGREDIENTS

tree peony bark, Cortex Moutan Radicis 12g

fresh—water turtle shell, Carapax Trionycis 50g

dried rehmannia root, Radix Rehmanniae 30g

PROCESS Decoct them together in water for oral administration.

DIRECTIONS To be taken 8 to 10 doses in succession, one dose a day.

3) Scales Glue (Yulin Jiao)

INGREDIENTS

scales of big fishes, such as black carp (Mylopharyngodon Aethops), Carp (Cyprinus Carpio), crucian carp (Carassius Auratus), right amount.

some seasonings:

yellow rice or millet wine

fresh ginger, Rhizoma Zingiberis Recens

table salt

gourmet powder

soy sauce

sesame oil, Oleum Sesami

PROCESS Wash the scales clean, boil them in water for 2 to 4 hours and strain the dregs out; then season them with the wine, fresh ginger, table salt and gourmet powder. They will become glue overnight.

DIRECTIONS Cut the glue into small pieces and mix them with soy sauce and sesame oil for eating. It is to be taken for several days running, once a day,350 to 400g each time.

Those who suffer from thrombopenic purpura marked by the tpye of interior heat due to yin—deficiency can select any of the above recipes for oral administration.

4)Soup of Wolfberry Fruit,Asia Bell,Chinese—Date and Egg(Gouqi Shen Zao Jidan Tang)

INGREDIENTS

wolfberry fruit,Fructus Lycii 10 to 15g

Chinese—date,Fructus Ziziphi Jujubae 10

Asia bell,Radix Codonopsis Pilosulae 15g

egg 2

PROCESS

Make soup with all the ingredients in an earthenware pot.

When the eggs are done,shell them and go on cooking for a few seconds.

DIRECTIONS The eggs are to be eaten and the soup to be drunk. It is to be taken 6 to 7 doses in succession,once a day or every other day. It is applicable to patients suffering from the type of failure of qi to keep the blood flowing in the vessels.

Section 29

Puerperal Hypogalactia

The morbid condition in which a parturient has scarce or no milk is called hypogalactia. Medicated dietetic therapy,has relatively good curative effects upon hypogalactia,in some cases,even can be used as a major therapy.

1. **Common Type of Syndromes**

1)One of the common syndromes is deficiency of both blood and qi Manifested as puerperal hypogalactia,soft mammae with no sensation of distending pain,pale complexion,loss of appetite,shortness of breath and lassitude,pale tongue with little fur,and soft and feeble pulse.

2)Another type is stagnation of the liver—qi Marked by galactostasis, feeling of distension, fullness and pain or having lumps in the mammae, sensation of fullness and distress in the chest and hypochondrium, poor appetite and hiccup, darkish red tongue, and taut and slippery pulse.

2. **Composite Recipes of Medicated Diet**

1) Soup of Fresh Mushroom for Nourishing the Spleen (Xianmo Yi Pi Tang)

INGREDIENTS

fresh mushroom, Agaricus Campestris (with caps torn into small pieces and stems cut into slanting slices) 100g

lean pork (cut into thin slices) 100g

PROCESS Stir—fry the meat in cooking oil and salt until it turns white, add just the right amount of water to boil the mushroom and meat until it is done, and then take it.

2) Soup of Black—bone Chicken (Wuji Tang)

INGREDIENTS

black—bone rooster, Gallus domesticus (cut into cubes) 1

dried orange peel, Pericarpium Citri Reticulatae 3g

galangal, Rhizoma Alpiniae Officinarum 3g

pepper, Fructus Piperis Nigri 6g

caoguo, Fructus Tsaoko 2

scallion and vinegar right amount each

PROCESS Have the black—bone rooster, the dried orange peel, galangal, pepper, caoguo, scallion and vinegar well—stewed, take the chicken with the soup.

3) Soup of Astragalus Root and Pork Liver (Huangqi Zhugan Tang)

INGREDIENTS

pork liver 500g

astragalus root, Radix Astragali seu Hedysari 60g

PROCESS Make soup with the pork liver and astragalus roots.

DIRECTIONS Take the liver and the soup.

Patients who have hypogalactia caused by deficiency of both qi and blood can choose one or two from the above recipes for oral use singly or together.

4) Recipe of Bean Curd, Towel Gourd, Mushroom and Pig's Trotter (Doufu Sigua Xianggu Ti)

INGREDIENTS

bean curd 500g

towel gourd ,Fructus Luffae(With its pulp) 250g

mushroom,Lentinus Edodes 50g

pig's trotter 1

Spices right amount

PROCESS Have the pig's and mushroom boiled together,flavour it with scallion,ginger and salt;after they are all done put in the towel gourd and bean curd to make soup.

DIRECTIONS Take it in three separate portions in one day. Take such soup for five days successively.

5)Recipe of Kelp,Finger Citron and Soy Bean Milk (Haidai Foshou Doujiang)

INGREDIENTS

soy bean milk,Succus Semi Sojae 500g

kelp,Thallus Laminariae 100g

finger citron,Fructus Citri Sarcodactylis 9g

PROCESS Make soup with the above ingredients and take it saltless , once a day for several days.

Patients who have hypogalactia caused by stagnation of the liver—qi can choose one or two for use from the above recipes.

Section 30

Mastitis

Acute mastitis is an acute inflammation caused by pyogenic germs invading mammary glands ,which is often evoked to rhagades of the nipple,deformed nipple,crater nipple and galactostasis. Breast—feeding women are most susceptible to the disease within one or two months after childbirth. Some unmarried women and ante—partum women may also get the disease, but the number is much smaller,whereas the incidence is relatively higher in primiparae. It is termed "ru yong"(acute mastitis) in traditional Chinese medicine.

1. **Common Type of Syndromes**

This disease is characterized by local red swelling in the breast accompanied with fever. Generally, it is treated as a disesae with abundant heat—toxin accumulated in the affected region in TCM.

The common type is caused by accumulation of abundant noxious heat, marked by local red swelling. If the swollen part is hard and has a pain when pressed and yet no apparent undulation, it shows no suppuration in this part; if there is apparent undulation with distending and throbbing pain, it means local abscess has formed. It is usually accompanied with symptoms such as fever, dry mouth and thirst, constipation, yellowish fur on the tongue and rapid pulse.

2. **Composite Recipes of Medicated Diet**

Decoction of Dandelion Herb and Honeysuckle Stem (Gonying Rendong Tang)

INGREDIENTS

dandelion herb, Herba Taraxaci 30g

honeysuckle stem, Caulis Lonicerae 30g

PROCESS Add the right amount of water and yellow rice(or millet) wine into 30g of dandelion herb and 30g of honeysuckle stem and decoct them together so as to get a thick extract. Drink it in two separate doses a day.

Section 31

Voice Disease

This disease is marked mainly by a hoarse voice. Medicated diet is of great benefit to the treatment of the disease.

1. **Common Types of Syndromes**

1) Stagnation of phlegm mingled with excessive heat Marked by a low and harsh voice, abundant, thick and yellowish phlegm, accompanied with bitter taste and dry throat, yellowish and greasy fur on the tongue, and slippery and rapid pulse.

2)Dryness of the lung and scanty body fluid Marked by a hoarse voice, gradual loss of voice, accompanied with dry mouth and pharynx, itching and pain in the throat, or dry cough, reddened tongue with scanty saliva, and thready and rapid pulse.

2. **Composite Recipes of Medicated Diet**

1)Decoction of Radish and Chinese Honey Locust(Luobu Zaojiao Tang)

INGREDIENTS

white radish, Radix Raphani 1 PC.

Chinese honey locust fruit, Fructus Gleditsiae 1. 5g

PROCESS Have the white radish cut into slices and decocted in water together with the Chinese honey locust fruit.

DIRECTIONS Drink the decoction and eat the radish.

It is applicable to patients with the type of stagnation of phlegm mingled with excessive heat.

2) Decoction of Scrophularia Root, Ophiopogon, Liquorice and Platycodon Root(Xuan Mai Gan Jie Tang)

INGREDIENTS

scrophularia root, Radix Scrophulariae 12g

ophiopogon, Radix Ophioponis 12g

platycodon root, Radix Platycodi 10g

liquorice, Radix Glycyrrhizae 3g

PROCESS Make decoction for oral administration with the above ingredients. It is applicable to cases with the type of dryness of the lung and scanty body fluid.

3)Gruel of Pear Juice(Lizhi Zhou)

INGREDIENTS

pear, Malum Piri 3 to 5

polished round—grained rice, Semen Oryzae Sativae 50g

crystal sugar right amount

PROCESS Have 3 to 5 pears washed clean, cut into pieces and pounded to get the juice; remove the dregs and put the juice, the polished round—grained rice and crystal sugar into an earthenware pot, add 400ml of water to make thin gruel.

DIRECTIONS Take it slightly warm two or three times a day. It has a remarkable effect of protecting and improving voice, especially for singers and announcers.

Section 32

Tonsillitis

This disease is termed "ru e" in traditional Chinese medicine.

1. **Common Type of Syndromes**

Accumulation of heat in the lung and stomach, and concurrent affecting exogenous pathogenic factors. Marked by a sudden high fever, swelling and pain or festering in the pharynx, restlessness, thirst and constipation, red tongue with thick and yellowish fur, and slippery and rapid pulse.

2. Composite Recipes of Medicated Diet

1) Cucumber Frost (Huanggua Shuang)

INGREDIENTS

ripe cucumber, Fructus Cucumeris Sativus 1

alum, Alumen a certain amount

PROCESS Get one big ripe cucumber, cut off its top end, remove the pulp and seeds, fill it up with alum, cover the cut end and fix it with a bamboo spike, put the cucumber in a string bag and hang it in a cool, shaded and ventilated place for several days until frost—like powder constantly oozes out through the skin of the cucumber, which is called "cucumber frost". Collect the powder by sweeping it down with a sterilized goose feather.

DIRECTIONS Gargle (with cold boiled water) after meals, and then have just the right amount of the "frost" blown onto the affected part (it can be swallowed down) at a time, several times a day, until the disease is cured.

2) Juices of Dayflower and Peppermint (Yazhi Bohezhi)

INGREDIENTS

dayflower, Herba Commelinae 120g

fresh peppermint, Herba Menthae 60g

PROCESS Have 120g of dayflower and 60g of fresh peppermint pounded into a mash and wrung to get the juices.

DIRECTIONS Take 30ml of the juice each time by keeping it in the mouth and swallowing it bit by bit at short intervals after mixing it thoroughly with the right amount of cold boiled water.

Section 33

Pharyngitis

Pharyngitis is divided into two kinds: acute and chronic. Acute pharyngitis, because of widespread red swelling in the part of throat, belongs to the category "houbi"(inflammation of the throat) in traditional Chinese medicine; while chronic pharyngitis belongs to the category of "meihe qi"(globus hystericus) because of apparent foreign body sensation in the part of throat. Medicated dietetic treatment is a desirable auxiliary aid to treating this disease.

1. **Common Types of Syndromes**

1) Invasion of the throat by wind—heat Marked by fever and chills at the onset, red swelling in the part of the pharynx, dry mouth with a feeling of burning, apparent pain and increasing secretion in the part of throat, headache and feeling of fullness in the head, red tongue with thin yellowish fur, and slippery and rapid pulse.

2) Impairment of the lung—yin due to lung heat Manifested as dryness and discomfort in the part of the pharynx, slight pain, apparent foreign body sensation, abundant and thick expectoration, deep—red tongue with little fur, and taut and rapid pulse; dark red retropharynx with bumps of lymph follicles can be seen when examined.

2. **Composite Recipes of Medicated Diet**

1) Drink of Radish and Chinese Olive (Luobo Ganlan Dai Cha Yin)

INGREDIENTS

radish, Napus 100g

Chinese olive, Fructus Canarin 30g

PROCESS Decoct the radish and Chinese olives in water to make decoction.

DIRECTIONS Take it as a drink, a dose a day, and 5 to 7 doses successively. It is applicable to the type of pharyngitis resulitng from wind—heat invading the pharynx.

2)Distillate of Scrophularia Root and Radish for Removing Pathogenic Heat from the Throat(Xuanshen Luobo Qing Ran Lu)

INGREDIENTS

white radish, Radix Raphani 300g

scrophularia root, Radix Scrophulariae 15g

arctium fruit, Fructus Arctii 15g

honey, Mel 80g

rice(or millet) wine 20ml

PROCESS Have the radish washed clean and cut into slices; have the scrophularia roots and arctium fruits washed clean and soaked in the wine for later use. Put a layer of radish slices in a porcelain basin, and on this layer, a layer of scrophularia roots and arctium fruits; drench them with about 10g of honey; put 4 or 5 layers this way; add 20ml of cold water into the remaining honey, and pour it into the porcelain basin. Steam the drugs over a brisk fire for two hours with the drugs not contacting water and then stop steaming.

DIRECTIONS Warm it up every day in a steamer for oral administration. Take it twice a day, 50ml of the distillate and 4 slices of radish at a time. It is applicable to patients suffering from the type of impairment of the lung—yin by lung—heat.

Section 34

Hemorrhoid

Hemorrhoid is an anal disease caused by varicose hemorrhoidal veins. There are internal hemorrhoid, external hemorrhoid and mixed hemorrhoid according to clinical manifestations. Medicated dietetic treatment has more desirable curative effect.

1. **Common Types of Syndromes**

1)The first type is blood stagnation At the inital stage of hemorrhoid, it is marked by mucosal congestion, discomfort with pruritus and to the accompaniment of foreign body sensation. It may cause a little bleeding and pain as a result of blood stagnation, dark red tongue, uneven pulse.

2)The second one is the damp—heat type Marked by a sensation of bearing—down, distending and burning pain in the anus, hematochezia, constipation or loose stool, scanty dark urine, dry mouth with bitter taste, red tongue with thick yellowish and greasy fur, wiry and rapid pulse.

3)The third one is the type of blood deficiency Marked by dizziness, tinnitus and pale complexion due to long—term hematochezia, pale tongue with thin whitish fur, and deep and thready pulse.

2. **Composite Recipes of Medicated Diet**

1)Decoction of Black Edible fungus(Heimuer Tang)

INGREDIENTS

black edible fungus, Auricularia 6g

dried persimmon, Fructus Kaki 50g

brown sugar 50g

PROCESS Decoct 6g of black edible fungus, 50g of dried persimmons and 50g of brown sugar together in water.

DIRECTIONS Take a dose daily for five to six days. This recipe is applicable to blood stagnation type.

2)Gruel of Mulberry(Sangshen Zhou)

INGREDIENTS

mulberry, Fructus Mori 20 to 30g

(or 30 to 60g if fresh)

polished glutinous rice, Semen Oryzae Glutinosae 100g

crystal sugar 25g

PROCESS First, submerge the mulberries in water for some time and wash them clean. Then, put them into an earthenware pot together with the glutinous rice to make gruel. Put in the crystal sugar and keep on cooking for a while.

DIRECTIONS Take it twice each day, on an empty stomach, and five to seven days making up a course of treatment.

It is applicable to the hemorrhoid of damp—heat type.

3)Recipe of Sea Cucumber and Donkey—hide Gelatin (Haishen Ejiao)

INGREDIENTS

sea cucumber, Stichopus Japonicus 15g

donkey—hide gelatin, Colla Corii Asini 6g

PROCESS Bake sea cucumbers till their outer parts become charred yet the inner parts are still yellowish—brown, so that their original porperty is retained. Grind them into fine powder. Stew 15g of the powder and 6g of donkey—hide gelatin together in 50 ml of water until the donkey—hide gelatin is dissolved.

DIRECTIONS It should be taken on an empty stomach with millet (or rice) water, three times a day, for four or five successive days. It is applicable to hemorrhoid of blood deficiency type.

Chapter Four

Medicated Diets for Nourishments and Longevity

Medicated diets for nourishment and longevity are all attached great importance by Chinese doctors of past ages. These doctors who have accumulated a wealth of experience and prescriptions of medicated diets consider these recipes as mainly used to treat various syndromes of debility as well as build up the physique for prolonging life.

Just as a renowned physician of the Tang Dynasty, Sun Simiao pointed out in Dietetic Therapy, a chapter of his book Prescriptions Worth A Thousand Gold for Emergencier, "Food can expel pathogenic factors from the human body, regulate the functions of the five viscera (the heart, liver, spleen, lung and kidney), please the senses, nourish the blood and invigorate qi", and Zhang Jiebin (1563—1640A. C.), a physician in the Ming Dynasty said "the creation of nourishing prescriptions is for deficiency syndromes. "Therefore medicated diets are classified into three groups according to their functions, that is, medicated diets for nourishing the blood, invigorating qi, strengthening yang and replenishing yin; medicated diets for tonifying the five viscera and medicated diets for improving the health and prolonging life.

Section 1

Medicated Diets for Nourishing Qi, Blood, Yin and Yang

1. Medicated Diets for Invigorating Qi

Medicated diets for invigorating qi are such foods cooked by mixing Chinese materia medica chosen for this purpose into certain foods. These medicated foods, having the function of invigorating qi , being able to enhance the resistance of organism and the function of immunity, build up the physique, increase the adaptability to the environment and strengthen the function of tissues and organs in the body, are applicable to syndromes of qi deficiency , marked by lassitude, deficiency of qi, disinclination to talk , dyspnea on slight exertion, sweating due to debility, liability to catching cold, pale complexion, inappetence , loose stool, pale or reddish tongue with white moist fur and feeble pulse.

1) Gruel for Restoring and Invigorating Qi (Buxu Zhengqi Zhou)

SOURCE General Collection For Holy Relief

INGREDIENTS

prepared astragalus root, Radix Astragali seu Hedysari 20g

dangshen, Radix Codonopsis Pilosulae 10g

polished round—grained rice, Semen Oryzae Sativae 100g

white sugar right amount

PROCESS Cut astragalus roots and dangshen into slices and soak them in clear water for 40 minutes , decoct them in water to get 30 ml of condensel extract. Make gruel with the washed rice; put in the condensed extract and go on cooking for a while.

DIRECTIONS Take it with as much white sugar as you think fit , twice a day , in the morning and in the evening respectively.

EFFICACY Invigorating the vital-qi, treating consumptive diseases and delaying senility.

INDICATIONS Impairment of the function of internal organs, emotional strain, infirmity due to old age, emaciation caused by prolonged illness, manifested as palpitation and shortness of breath, weakness, spontaneous perspiration, inappetence, protracted diarrhea due to insufficiency of the spleen, and so on.

PRECAUTIONS Generally, eat such gruel for 3 to 5 days successively, resume eating 2 to 3 days later. Radish and tea are prohibited during the period of taking such gruel.

2) Soup of Ginseng and Lotus Seed Kernel (Renshen Lianrou Tang)

SOURCE proved Effective Prescriptions

INGREDIENTS

white ginseng, Radix Ginseng 10g

lotus seed, Semen Nelumbinis 10g

crystal sugar 30g

PROCESS Put white ginseng and lotus seeds (rid of the lotus plumules) in a bowl, add the right amount of clean water to make them expand by soaking, then, add the crystal sugar. Put the bowl with the drugs in a steamer to steam without its contacting water for an hour. The ginseng can be used three times successively——add lotus seed kernels, crystal sugar and the right amount of water the following day to make soup in the same way.

DIRECTIONS Drink the soup and eat the lotus seed kernels; at the third time, eat the ginseng as well. Take it twice a day, once in the morning and in the evening respectively.

EFFICACY Invigorating qi and replenishing the spleen.

INDICATIONS Symptoms after an illness such as weakness, deficiency of qi, anorexia, lassitude, spontaneous perspiration; or diarrhea due to deficiency of the spleen.

PRECAUTIONS It is prohibited to use an ironware to make the soup and take radish and tea.

3) Chicken Stewed with Astragalus Root (Huangqi Qiguo Ji)

SOURCE Cookbook of Suiyuan

INGREDIENTS

young hen 1

astragalus root, Radix Astragali seu Hedysari 30g
refined salt 5g
cooking wine 15g
scallion, Bulbus Allii fistulosi 10g
fresh ginger, Rhizoma Zingiberis Recens 10g
gourmet powder right amount
pepper powder, Pulvis Fruclus Piperis right amount

PROCESS Kill the hen, remove its feathers, cut off its claws, get rid of its internal organs, wash it clean and scald it in boiling water until the folds on the skin spread out;、wash it in cold water and drain; have the astragalus roots washed clean and cut into sections 6 to 7 cm long (each cut lengthwise into halves); then, put them tidily in the chicken's abdominal cavity; have the scallion and ginger washed clean and cut into sections and slices respectively; put the chicken in a small food steamer, add the scallion sections, ginger slices, cooking wine, and salt; cover the steamer tight, then, put it in a big food steamer and heat it over a strong fire to boiling point for about two hours. After taking it out from the big steamer, pick the scallion and ginger out; then, take the astragalus roots out from the chicken's abdominal cavity, stack them on the chicken, season it with pepper powder before eating.

DIRECTIONS It can be taken with bread or cooked rice.

EFFICACY Replenishing qi and elevating yang; nourishing the blood and treating syndromes of deficiency.

INDICATIONS Anorexia due to deficiency of the spleen, weakness, spontaneous perspiration, liability to catching cold caused by deficiency of qi; dizziness due to deficiency of blood; prolapse of rectum, prolonged diarrhea, prolapse of uterus and other symptoms resulting from sinking of qi of the middle—jiao. It can be used as health—improving food for those who are weak after an illness and for those who suffer from malnutrition, anemia, nephritis and prolapse of internal organs. As for those who are healthy, it can be used to build up their physique and prevent them from catching cold if taken often.

2. Medicated Diets for Nourishing the Blood

Medicated diets for nourishing the blood are cooked by mixing Chinese materia medica chosen for this purpose into certain foods. They have the effects of nourishing the blood and the liver, replenishing the heart and spleen, and are applicable to deficiency of blood, marked by giddiness, lassitude, numblimbs, palpitaion or severe palpitation, insomnia, amnesia, sallow complexion, pale lips and tongue and nails, and thready and rapid or thready and uneven pulse.

1) Thick Soup of Chinese Angelica Root and Mutton (Danggui Yangrou Geng)

SOURCE Prescriptions for Succouring the Sick

INGREDIENTS

Chinese angelica root, Radix Angelicae Sinensis 15g

astragalus roots, Radix Astragali seu Hedysari 25g

dangshen, Radix Codonopsis Pilosulae 25g

mutton 500g

scallion, fresh ginger, cooking wine and gourmet powder right amount for each

PROCESS Wash the mutton clean; put Chinese Angelica roots, astragalus roots and dangshen into a gauze bag and tie up its opening; put scallion, ginger, salt and cooking wine together into an aluminium pan, add the right amount of water. Heat it over a strong fire to boiling point, change to stewing it gently over a low fire until the mutton is thoroughly done. Add gourmet powder before eating.

DIRECTIONS Eat the mutton and drink the soup, twice a day, once in the morning and in the evening respectively.

EFFICACY Nourishing the blood and treating syndromes of deficiency.

INDICATIONS Deficiency of blood or weakness after an illness of delivery manifested as abdominal cold—pain, cold sensation in uterus with blood deficiency, metrorrhagia or metrostaxis and other kinds of anemia.

PRECAUTIONS Those who have a fever due to exopathy, painful swelling in the throat and toothache are prohibited to take such soup. It is prohibited to use a copper ware and to eat pumpkin.

2) Recipe of Chinese Angelica Root, Dangshen, Chinese Yam and Pig Kidney (Gui Shen Shanyao Zhuyao)

SOURCE Select Recipes of 100

INGREDIENTS

Chinese angelica root, Radix Angelicae Sinensis 10g

dangshen, Radix Codonopsis Pilosulae 10g

Chinese yam, Rhizoma Dioscoreae 10g

pig kidney 500g

soy sauce, vineger, shredded ginger, mashed garlic, sesame oil just the right amount for each

PROCESS　Cut the pigs kidney open, remove the fasciae and the renal pelvis, and wash it clean; put Chinese angelica open and put it together with the pigs kidney in an aluminium pan; add just the right amount of water, have the ingredients boiled in clear soup (without soy sauce) until the pig kidney is well done. Take the kidney out and let it cool. Cut it into thin slices, put it on a plate and then mix it with soy sauce, vinegar, shredded ginger, mashed garlic and sesame oil.

DIRECTIONS　Take it with bread or cooked rice.

EFFICACY　Nourishing the blood, replenishing qi and invigorating the kidney.

INDICATIONS　Palpitaion, shortness of breath, pain and soreness of waist, insomnia, spontaneous perspiration and other symptoms due to deficiency of qi and blood accompanied with deficiency of the kidney.

3. Medicated Diets for Nourishing Yin

The medicated diets for nourishing yin are cooked by mixing Chinese materia medica chosen for this purpose into certain foods. They have the effects of nourishing yin and tonifying the kidney, replenishing the vital essence to promote the generatic of marrow, and are applicable to deficiency of yin, manifested as emaciation, giddiness, dry mouth and throat, insomnia due to vexation, hectic fever, night perspiration, redness in the zygomatic region, red lips, dysphoria with feverish sensation in the chest, palms and soles, lassitude in the loins and knees, emission, forgetfulness, reddened tongue with little fur, and thready and rapid pulse.

1) Gruel with Lucid Asparagus Root (Tianmendong Zhou)

SOURCE　Collection of Selected Diets

INGREDIENTS

lucid asparagus root, Radix Asparagi 15 to 20g

polished round-grained rice, Semen Oryzae Sativae 60g

crystal sugar right amount

PROCESS　First, decoct lucid asparagus roots in water to get concentrated extract, remove the dregs; put in the polished round—grained rice to make gruel; add crystal sugar after it has boiled and go on cooking for a while.

DIRECTIONS Take the gruel once in the morning and once in the evening respectively.

EFFICACY Replenishing the vital essence and moisturizing the lung, and promoting production of the body fluid to quench thirst.

INDICATIONS Interior heat syndrome due to deficiency of the kidney—yin, marked by dry mouth and hypoptyalism; heat syndrome caused by deficiency of the lung—yin, manifested as dry cough with little or no sputum, sputum mixed with blood; pulmonary tuberculosis with symptoms of low fever in the afternoon and night sweating.

PRECAUTIONS Take such gruel for 3 to 5 days as a course of treatment; resume taking it three days later; those who suffer from abdominal pain due to cold of deficiency type, cough due to affection by wind—cold should not take such gruel.

2) Specially—prepared Black Soybean (Fazhi Heidou)

SOURCE Complete Works of Zhang Jingyue

INGREDIENTS

black soybean, Semen Sojae Nigrum 500g

dogwood fruit, Fructus Corni 10g

poria, Poria 10g

Chinese angelica root, Radix Angelicae Sinsis 10g

mulberry, Fructus Mori 10g

prepared rehmannia root, Radix Rehmanniae Praeparata 10g

psoralea fruit, Fructus Psoraleae 10g

dodder seed, Semen Cuscutae 10g

eclipta, Herba Ecliptae 10g

schisandra fruit, Fructus Schisandrae 10g

wolfberry fruit, Fructus Lycii 10g

wolfberry bark, Cortex Lycii Radicis 10g

sesame seed, Semen Sesami Nigrum 10g

salt, Sal Communis

PROCESS Soak the black soybeans in lukewarm water for 30 minutes; put the other drugs listed above (except the salt) into a gauze bag, tie it up, then, put it in an aluminium pan; add just the right amount of water to heat it; take out decoction once every 30 minutes and put it in a basin; add water into the aluminium pan to heat it again; thus, make and take out decoction four times altogether; put all the decoction into the aluminium pan. Put black soybeans into the pan containing the decoction and put in the salt; heat it over a strong fire until the decoction has boiled, then change to a low fire until decoction has run dry. Dry the black soybeans in the sun. Put the black soybeans into a china pot (or a bottle) for later use.

DIRECTIONS Chew as many as your appetite permits.

EFFICACY Tonifying and replenishing the vital essence of the kidney to strengthen the muscles and bones.

INDICATIONS Giddiness, tinnitus, deafness, emaciation, frequent micturitio, emission, soreness in the loins and pain in the legs, flaccidity of extremities and other symptoms caused by insufficiency of the vital essence of the kidney and deficiency of the kidney—yin.

4. **Medicated Diets for Restoring Yang**

Medicated diets for restoring yang are those cooked by mixing warm—natured drugs chosen for this purpose into certain foods. They have the effects of warming the kidney, invigorating yang, strengthening the constitution, exciting sexuality, enhancing sexual function and genitality, and are applicable to deficiency of yang——mainly that of both the spleen and the kidney, manifested as tinnitus, giddiness, lassitude or cold—pain in the loins and knees, impotence premature ejeculation, sterility in women, clear urine, loose stool, pale complexion, listlessness, pale tongue, and deep, thready and feeble pulse.

1) Gruel with Desertliving Cistanche and Mutton (Congrong Yangrou Zhou)

SOURCE Compendium of Materia Medica

INGREDIENTS

desertliving cistanche, Herba Cistanchis 10 to 15g
chosen mutton 60g
polished round—grained rice, Semen Oryzae Sativae 60g
refined salt, Sal Communis a bit
scallion stalks, Bulbus Allii Fistulosi (cut into slices) 2
fresh ginger, Rhizoma Zingiberis Recens 3 slices

PROCESS Have desertliving cistanche and chosen mutton washed clean and cut into slices; first, decoct the desertliving cistanche in an earthenware pot to obtain extract and remove the dregs; then, put in the mutton and the rice; add salt, scallion stalks and fresh ginger into the pot to make thin gruel.

DIRECTIONS Take such gruel once in the morning and once in the evening.

EFFICACY Replenishing the kidney, invigorating yang, improving the function of the spleen, tonifying the stomach and loosening the bowel to relieve constipation.

INDICATIONS Insufficiency of the kidney—yang, manifested as impotence, emission, premature ejeculation, sterility in women, cold—pain in the loins and knees, frequent micturition, polyuria at night, general debility, internal injury due to overstrain, chills and intolerance of cold, cold limbs, cold of deficiency type in the spleen and stomach, and constipation due to insufficiency of yang in the aged.

PRECAUTIONS Gruel with desertliving cistanche and mutton is warm—natured medicated gruel, fit to be taken in winter; take it for 5 to 7 days as a course of treatment; those who suffer from loose stool, sexual hyperesthesia, should not take it; it is not fit to be taken in summer.

2) Dog Meat Soup for Promoting Yang(Zhuang Yang Gourou Tang)

SOURCE Popular Medicated Diets

INGREDIENTS

prepared aconite root, Radix Aconiti Praeparata(cut into slices) 15g

dodder seed, Semen Cuscutae 10g

dog meat 250g

salt, gourmet powder, fresh giner, scallion

just the right amount for each

PROCESS Have the dog meat washed clean, put it as one piece into a pot with boiling water and quick—boil it through; take it out and put it into cold water to remove the blood froth; and cut it into cubes. Cut fresh ginger and scallion into slices; stirfry the dog meat in an aluminium pan together with ginger slices; pour it into an earthenware pot after adding cooking wine; meanwhile, put the dodder seeds and the prepared aconite roots slices in a gauze bag and tie it up; put the bag together with salt and scallion into the earthenware pot; add just the right amount of clear soup which is heated to boiling point over a strong fire, then, change to stewing it on a low fire until the dog's meat is thoroughly done. Add gourmet powder before eating.

DIRECTIONS　Eat the meat and drink the soup; it can be taken with bread or cooked rice.

EFFICACY　Warming the kidney, recuperating the kidney—yang and replenishing the essence to nourish the marrow.

INDICATIONS　Deficiency of yang and qi, marked by listlessness, lassitude in the loins and knees , etc.

PRECAUTIONS　Those who suffer from deficiency of yin are prohibited to take it.

5. **Medicated Diets for Replenishing All of Qi, Blood, Yin and Yang**

These medicated diets are cooked by mixing Chinese materia medica chosen for tonifying qi and yang, replenishing yin and nourishing blood into certain foods. They have the effects of recuperating both qi and blood, tonifying yin and warming yang, replenishing essence and nourishing marrow, and are applicable to deficiency of qi, blood, yin and yang, which is manifested as shortness of breath, disinclination to talk, listlessness, dizziness and palpitation, spontaneous perspiration or night sweating, hectic fever or intolerance to cold, cold limbs, etc.

1) Decoction of Ten Powerful Tonics (Shi Quan Da Bu Tang)

SOURCE　Popular Medicated Diets

INGREDIENTS

dangshen, Radix Codonopsis Pilosulae 10g

prepared astragalus root, Radix Astragali seu Hedysari 10g

Chinese cassia tree bark, Cortex Cinnamomi 3g

prepared rehmannia root, Radix Rehmanniae Praeparata 15g

parched bighead atractylodes rhizome, Rhizoma Atractylodis Macrocephalae 10g

parched chuanxiong rhizome, Rhizoma Ligustici Chuanxiong 6g

Chinese angelica root, Radix Angelicae Sinensis 15g

wine—steeped white peony root, Radix Paeoniae Alba 10g

poria, Poria 10g

prepared liquorice, Radix Glycyrrhizae 6g

inkfish, Sepia 50g

pork 500g

pork tripe 50g

fresh ginger, Rhizoma Zingiberis Recens 30g

pork bones, green Chinese onion (or scallion),

cooking wine, salt, Chinese prickly ash,

gourmet powder just the right amount of each

PROCESS Put the above medicinal herbs into a clean gauze bag and tie up the opening for later use; have the pork, inkfish and pork tripe washed clean, pork bones washed clean and cracked by pounding, fresh ginger beaten into pieces, and put them together with the medicinal herb bag into an aluminium pan; add just the right amount of water, put in Chinese prickly ash, cooking wine and salt, then, heat the pan over a strong fire until the water has boiled; change to stewing it over a low fire. When the pork is thoroughly done, take it out and cut it into short thin pieces, then place it back into the decoction and remove the medicinal herb bag.

DIRECTIONS Take it twice in a day, once in the morning and once in the evening; eat the meat and drink the decoction.

EFFICACY Replenishing both qi and blood.

INDICATIONS Deficiency of both qi and blood or debility after a protracted illness, manifested as sallow complexion, listlessness, lassitude in the loins and knees, etc.

PRECAUTIONS Resume taking it five days after the first treatment. Those suffering from common cold of wind—cold type are prohibited to take it.

2) Gruel of "Pearl and Jade" (Zhu Yu Er Bao Zhou)

SOURCE Records of Traditional Chinese and Western Medicine in Combination

INGREDIENTS

raw Chinese yam, Rhizoma Dioscoreae 60g

coix seed, Semen Coicis 60g

cake of frostlike powder on the surface of dried

persimmon, Mannosum Kaki 24g

PROCESS First, have Chinese yam and coix seeds pounded into coarse pieses and cooked until they are thoroughly done; then, cut the cake of dried persimmon frost into small pieces and mix them into the gruel and wait for them to dissolve.

DIRECTIONS Take it twice a day, once in the morning and once in the evening.

EFFICACY Replenishing the spleen and the lung, and removing heat from them; tonifying and moistening yin with drugs sweet in taste and moist in nature.

INDICATIONS Anorexia, low fever in the afternoon, or even hectic fever and night sweating, cough especially at night, hollow, rapid and taut pulse caused by deficiency of qi and yin of the spleen and lung.

Section 2

Medicated Diets for Tonifying and Benefiting Five Viscera

1. Medicated Diets for Strengthening the Spleen

Medicated diets for strengthening the spleen are cooked by mixing some materia medica chosen for invigorating the spleen and nourishing qi into certain foods. They have the effects of invigorating the spleen, nourishing qi, normalizing the function of the stomach and regulating qi of the middle—jiao(TCM holds it is the part where the spleen and stomach lie). They are applicable to deficiency of the spleen and weakness of qi, manifested as listlessness, lassitude of limbs, shortness of breath and disinclination to talk, dizziness, spontaneous perspiration, loss of appetite, dull pain in the stomach, loose stool, pale tongue with whitish fur, and relaxed and feeble pulse.

1)Cooked Rice with Dangshen and Chinese Dates(Shen Zao Mifen)

SOURCE Recipe of Xingyuan

INGREDIENTS

danshen, Radix Codonopsis Pilosulae 10g

Chinese—date, Fructus Ziziphi Jujubae 20g

polshed logn—grained glutinous rice, Semen Oryzae Glutionosae 250g white sugar 50g

PROCESS　Put dangshen and Chinese—dates in an earthenware pot, add water to make them expand. Decoct them in water for about 30 minutes and take out dangshen and Chinese—dates; wash the glutinous rice clean, put it in a big porcelain bowl with just the right amount of water and steam until the rice is done. Turn the bowl upside down to put the cooked rice on a plate. Put dangshen and Chinese-dates on the rice. Add white sugar into the prepared extract of dangshen and Chinese—dates and concentrate it, then, pour it on the cooked Chinese—date rice.

DIRECTIONS　It can be taken for breakfast.

EFFICACY　Strengthening the spleen and nourishing qi.

INDICATIONS　Deficiency of qi due to weak consititution, manifested as lassitude, palpitation, insomnia, loss of appetite, loose stool, dropsy, etc.

2) Gruel with Ginseng and Poria (Shen Ling Zhou)

SOURCE　General Collection for Holy Relief

INGREDIENTS

ginseng, Radix Ginseng 3 to 5g (or 15 to 20g of dangshen)

poria, Poria 15 to 20g

fresh ginger, Rhizoma Zingiberis Recens 3 to 5g

polished round—grained rice, Semen Oryzae Sativae 60g

PROCESS　Have the ginseng (or dangshen) and fresh ginger cut into thin slices, poria pounded into pieces. After soaking them for half an hour, decoct them in water for 30 minutes. Take out the extract and go on decocting it to obtain extract again. Put together the two extracts. Wash rice clean and put it into the extract to make gruel.

DIRECTIONS　Take such gruel once in the morning and once in the evening.

EFFICACY　Invigorating the middle—jiao and replenishing qi, strengthening the spleen and regulating the stomach.

INDICATIONS　Deficiency of qi, weak constitution and insufficiency of the spleen and stomach, manifested as lassitude, pale complexion, poor appetite, regurgitation and vomiting, loose stool, etc.

2. **Medicated Diets for Tonifying the Lung**

Medicated diets for nourishing the lung are cooked by mixing materia medica chosen for recuperating the lung—qi, nourishing yin and moistening the lung into certain foods. They have the effects of tonifying the lung—qi, nourishing yin, moistening the lung and arresting cough, and are applicable to insufficiency of the lung—qi or deficiency of the lung—yin. Insufficiency of the lung—qi is manifested as shortness of breath, disinclination to talk, cough with thin and clear sputum, preference for warmth, spontaneous sweating , susceptibility to cold, pale complexion; while deficiency of the lung—yin is marked by cough, dry cough with no or little and sticky sputum, emaciation, tidal fever in the afternoon, night sweating, flushing of zygomatic regions, etc.

1)Gruel with Lily Bulb (Baihe Zhou)

SOURCE Collection of Selected Diets

INGREDIENTS

fresh lily bulbs ,Bulbus Lilii Recens 30 to 50g

polished round—grained rice, Semen Oryzae Sativae 50g

crystal sugar right amount

PROCESS Have the rice washed clean and put it in a cooking pot; add just the right amount of water and heat it over a strong fire until it boils; change it to a low fire and heat it 40 minutes; put in the lily bulbs and go on cooking until it is done. Add crystal sugar before eating.

DIRECTIONS Take such gruel once in the morning and once in the evening.

EFFICACY Recuperating the lung, nourishing the spleen and relieving asthma and cough.

INDICATIONS Deficiency of the lung—yin and weakness of the spleen—qi, manifested as dry cough, asthma, lassitude, inappetence, fever of deficiency type and fidgetiness at times.

2) Stewed Whole Duck with Chinese Caterpillar Fungus (Chongcao Quanya)

SOURCE Supplement to the Compendium of Materia Medica

INGREDIENTS

Chinese caterpillar fungus, Cordyceps 10g

old drake 1

cooking wine 15g

fresh ginger, Rhizoma Zingiberis Recens 5g

scallion stalk, Bulbus Allii Fistulosi 10g

pepper powder, Pulvis Fructus Piperis Albi 3g

salt, Sal Communis 3g

PROCESS Have the drake killed and get rid of its feathers; cut off its webbed feed and cut its belly open to remove its internal organs; after washing it clean, scald it in a cooking pot with boiling water for a while; take it out and wash it clean with cold water. Wash the Chinese caterpillar fungus to remove mud and sand; have the scallion stalk and fresh ginger washed clean and cut into slices for later use. Cut the drake's head open along its neck, put 8 to 10 Chinese caterpillar fungi into the drake's head, tie it up tight with cotton thread; put the remaining fungi together with fresh ginger and scallion into the drake's abdomen; put the drake in a small pot, pour some water into it, add salt, pepper powder and cooking wine to season it, cover the pot closely with damp soft paper; steamer it in a bamboo steamer for about one and a half hours. Take the drake out from the steamer, remove the paper, pick the scallion and fresh ginger out, then, add gourmet powder to season it.

DIRECTIONS Eat the drake and drink the soup with bread (or cooked rice).

EFFICACY Replenishing the lung and kidney, tonifying the vital essence, nourishing marrow, arresting cough and relieving asthma.

INDICATIONS Asthma, cough, spontaneous sweating, impotence and emission caused by deficiency of the lung—qi or deficiecny of both the lung and the kidney, and weakness, listlessness, anorexia after an illness.

3. Medicated Diets for Nourishing the Heart

Medicated diets for nourishing the heart are cooked by mixing medicinal herbs chosen for nourishing the heart and tranquilizing the mind into certain foods. They have the effect of nourishing the heart—blood, replenishing the heart—qi, tranquilizing the mind, and benefiting the mental power, and are applicable to symptoms caused by deficiency of blood and qi of the heart such as palpitation, shortness of breath, depressed chest, palpitation on slight exertion, insomnia, excessive dreaming in sleep, failing memory, etc.

1) Gruel of Longan Aril (Longyanrou Zhou)

SOURCE Common Saying for Senile Health Preservation

INGREDIENTS

longan aril, Arillus Longan 15g

jujube, Fructus Ziziphi Jujubae 3 to 5

polished round-grained rice, Semen Oryzae Sativae 60g

PROCESS Have the rice washed clean, longan arils and jujubes washed off mud and sand; cook them together to make gruel.

DIRECTIONS Take such gruel once in the morning and once in the evening.

EFFICACY Nourishing the heart, tranquilizing the mind, strengthening the spleen and recuperating the blood.

INDICATIONS Palpitation, insomnia, forgetfulness and anemia caused by deficiency of the heart-blood; diarrhea, dropsy and constitutional frailty due to deficiency of the spleen; neurosism, spontaneous sweating and night sweating.

PRECAUTIONS The amount to be used should not be too great. It should be taken hot; prohibited to take such gruel are those who have common cold due to affection by pathogenic wind and cold, marked by fever and chills or thick and greasy fur on the tongue.

2) Stewed Pork Heart with Arborvitae Seed (Baiziren Dun Zhuxin)

SOURCE Popular Medicated Diets

INGREDIENTS

arborvitae seed, Semen Biotae 15g

pork heart 1

PROCESS Wash the pork heart clean and cut it open with a thin piece of bamboo; put the arborvitae seeds into the pork heart, and then put it in an earthenware pot and add just the right amount of water to stew it without its contacting water until it is thoroughly done.

DIRECTIONS Eat the heart and drink the soup.

EFFICACY Nourishing the heart and tranquilizing the mind, replenishing the blood and moistening the intestines.

INDICATIONS Palpitation, insomnia, excessive dreaming during sleep and failing memory due to deficiency of the heartblood and the heart-yin; constipation and other symptoms due to deficiency of blood in old age.

4. **Medicated Diets for Tonifying the Kidney**

Medicated diets for nourishing the kidney are cooked by mixing Chinese materia medica chosen for replenishing the kidney-qi, warming the kidney-yang, tonifying the kidney—yin into certain foods. They have the effects of warming the kidney, strengthening yang, replenishing the vital essence and promoting the generation of marrow, and are applicable to syndromes such as deficiency of the kidney including deficiency of the kidney—yin and kidney—yang, manifested as lassitude in the loins and knees, dizziness and tinnitus, insomnia, forgetfulness, emission and frequent urine, tidal fever, night sweating, dry mouth, or intolerance of cold, cold limbs and asthma.

1)Pill of Dodder Seed(Tusizi Wan)

SOURCE Food and Treatment of Diseases

INGREDIENTS

dodder seed, Semen Cuscutae 150g

poria, Poria 100g

lotus fruit pulp, Semen Nelumbinis 60g

PROCESS Grind the three drugs into fine powder; beat it with rice (or millet) wine to make paste, and then make it into pills the size of a Chinese parasol seed. Keep the pills in a bottle for later use.

DIRECTIONS Take 30 to 50 pills (about 9 to 12g) at a time, twice a day, once in the morning and once in the evening.

EFFICACY Nourishing the kidney and reinforcing the urinary bladder.

INDICATIONS Deficiency of the kidney—qi and hypofunction of the urinary bladder, manifested as enuresis accompanied with soreness of waist, frequent micturition, incontinence of urine and dribbling urination in cold weather but no burning pain sensation in the urethra.

2)Fried Duck with Walnut(Hetao Yazi)

SOURCE Imitated Court Menu

INGREDIENTS

walnut kernal, Semen Juglandis 200g

water chestnut, Bulbus Heleocharis Tuberosae 150g

old duck 1

minced chicken 100g

minced rape, scallion, fresh ginger, salt, egg white, cooking wine, corn flour paste, gourmet powder and peatnut oil right amount each

PROCESS Have the duck killed, remove its feathers, cut open its belly to remove its internal organs, wash it clean and then, quick—boil it in boiling water;

put it in a basin, add a bit of scallion, fresh ginger, salt and cooking wine; steam it in a cooking steamer until the duck is thoroughly done; take it out and let it cool, remove its bones and cut it into halves; make paste by mixing the minced chicken, egg white, corn flour paste , gourmet powder, cooking wine and salt, put the minced walnut kernel and water chestnuts into the paste, then, spread the paste over the inside wall of the duck's chest. Pour cooking oil into a pan, put in the duck when the oil is hot and fry it in deep oil until it becomes crisp. Take the duck out and let the remaining oil drip from the duck. Then, cut it into long cubes and have them arranged on a plate , spread some minced rape around the duck.

'DIRECTIONS Take it as dishes.

EFFICACY Replenishing the kidney and arresting seminal emission, warming the lung to relieve asthma, loosening the bowel to relieve constipation.

INDICATIONS Deficiency of the kidney , manifested as cough, pain in the waist, impotence, seminal emission, constipation, stranguria caused by the passage of urinary stone.

5. **Medicated Diets for Benefiting the Liver**

Medicated diets for benefiting the liver are cooked by mixing Chinese materia medica chosen for nourishing the liver and blood , improving acuity of vision, calming the endopathic wind and checking exuberance of yang into certain foods. They have the effects of nourishing the liver and blood, improving acuity of vision and concurrently nourishing the kidney , checking exuberance of yang, tranquilizing the mind, and are applicable to stirring up of endopathic wind of deficiency type caused by excess of yang due to deficiency of the liver-blood and liver—yin , manifested as giddiness, dim vision, or distending pain, dryness and discomfort of the eyes , hot temper and irritability, pain in the hypochondria, numbness of hands and feet, or even hemiplegia, and taut, thready and rapid pulse.

1)Goat(or Sheep)Liver Soup(Siwu Ganpian Tang)

SOURCE Dieteitc health—Preserving Recipe

INGREDIENTS

goat(or sheep)liver 200g

prepared rehmannia root, Radix Rehmanniae Praeparata 10g

chuanxiong rhizome, Rhizoma Ligustici Chuanxiong 3g

Chinese angelica root, Radix Angelicae Sinensis 6g

white peony root, Radix Paeoniae Alba 8g

wolfberry fruit, Fructus Lycii 10g
eclipta, Herba Ecliptae 6g
parched wild jujube seed, Semen Ziziphi Spinosae 6g
peper powder, Pulvis Fructus Piperis Albi 1g
gourmet powder 2g
soaked edible fungus, Auricularia 20g
cooking wine 2g
day lily, Flos Hemerocallis Immaturus 10g
wet starch 20g
chicken broth 400g
refined salt 6g
soy sauce 3g

PROCESS Wash the above medicinal herbs clean and put them into an earthenware pot; add water to decoct them for decoction and let the decoction settle to remove the sediment. Wash the goat liver clean, cut it into thin slices and put it into a bowl; add 2g of refined salt, soy sauce, cooking wine and wet starch and mix them thoroughly. Put the earthenware pot with the decoction in it over a strong fire, add chicken broth, edible fungus and day lily. When the decoction boils, take the edible fungus and day lily out and put them in a soup bowl. Spread the liver slices into the pot; skim off the froth when it boils again; put in salt, pepper powder, prepared lard and gourmet powder when the liver is done. Then, put it into the soup bowl for taking.

DIRECTIONS It can be taken with bread (or cooked rice).

EFFICACY Nourishing the liver, replenishing the blood, improving acuity of vision and tranquilizing the mind.

INDICATIONS Night blindness, dim eyesight and opticatrophy caused by deficiency of the liver—blood, palpitation, insomnia, forgetfulness and, in women, irregular menstruation, and other symptoms resulting from deficiency of the heart—blood.

6. Medicated Diets for Invigorating All the Viscera

Medicated diets for invigorating all the viscera are cooked by mixing Chinese materia medica chosen for replenishing the five viscera and treating consumptive diseases into certain foods. This category of medicated foods has the effects of replenishing deficiency, nourishing qi and blood, and tonifying the five viscera, and therefore, is capable of improving nutrition, strengthening the immunologic function of organism and disease—resistance, which results in improving health, tranquilizing the mind, stimulating the appetite and exciting sexual function. It is applicable to all syndromes of deficiency, manifested as emaciation, malnutrition, pale complexion, palpitation, shortness of breath, insomnia, forgetfulness, lassitude and poor appetite, low fever due to consumptive diseases, constipation, etc.

1)Gruel with Arborvitae Seed (Baiziren Zhou)

SOURCE　Gruel Menu

INGREDIENTS

arborvitae seed, Semenn Biotae 10 to 15g

honey, Mel right amount

polished round—grained rice, Semen Oryzae Sativae 30 to 60g

PROCESS　First , remove the shell and impurities of arborvtae seeds, pound them a bit and use them to make gruel together with rice. Add honey when the gruel is about to be done and go on cooking until it has boiled once or twice.

DIRECTIONS　Take such gruel once in the morning and once in the evening, for two or three days as a course of treatment.

EFFICACY　Nourishing the five viscera and strengthening the constitution, tonifying the heart and moistening the intestines.

INDICATIONS　Constipation, palpitation, insomnia and forgetfulness caused by weak constitution and dryness of the intestines.

PRECAUTIONS　For the old and the weak, walnut kernel should be used instead of honey. Persons who suffer from loose stool amd have a fever are prohibited to take it.

2)Soup of Sheep (or Goat)Viscera (Yangzang Geng)

SOURCE　Principles of Correct Diet

INGREDIENTS

sheep liver 1

sheep tripe 1

sheep heart 1

sheep lungs a set

sheep kidneys a pair

long pepper, Fructus Piperis Longi 50g

tsaoko cardamon, Fructus Tsaoko 2

dried orange peel, Pericarpium Citru Reticulatae 10g

lard, Lardum 50g

pepper Fructus Piperis 50g

fresh ginger, Rhizoma Zingiberis Recens 10g

scallion, Bulbus Allii Fistulosi 10g

fermented bean, Semen Sojae Fermentum 150g

salt, gourmet powder and cooking wine right amount each

PROCESS Have the sheep liver, heart, lungs, and kidneys washed clean, get rid of blood and water, and cut into cubes 2 cm^3; put long pepper, tsaoko cardamon, orange peel, pepper, ginger, scallion and fermented soybens into a gauze bag and tie it up tight; insert the bag into the sheep tripe; put the tripe together with the other viscera in an aluminium pan after sewing the tripe up; add just the right amount of water and put in the lard and salt. Heat the pan over a strong fire until the water boils, and then change to stewing it gently over a low fire until the contents are well done; take the sheep tripe out, remove the thread and take the medicinal bag out, cut the sheep tripe, heart, liver, lung and kidney into small cubes and put them back into the soup. Heat it again until it boils.

DIRECTIONS It can be taken with bread (or cooked rice).

EFFICACY Tonifying the five viscera and replenishing vital essence and qi.

INDICATIONS Deficiency of the five viscera and general asthenia.

Section 3

Medicated Diets for Prolonging Life

This group of medicated diets are cooked by mixing some Chinese materia medica chosen for improving health, strengthening the body resistance and consolidating the constitution into certain foods. They have the effects of regulating yin and yang, replenishing qi and blood, improving the function of the spleen, tonifying the kidney and nourishing essence, and are capable of lowering cholesterol, maintaining the elasticity of blood vessels, regulating blood pressure, increasing the immunologic function of organism, preventing diseases from occuring and prolonging life. They are applied to people of all ages, especially to those of the middle—aged and the old.

1) Medicinal Gruel with Sparrow (Queer Yao Zhou)

SOURCE Peaceful Holy Benevolent Prescriptions

INGREDIENTS

sparrow, Passer Montanus saturatus 5

dodder seed, Semen Cuscutae 30 to 45g

raspberry, Fructus Rubi 10 to 15g

wolfberry fruit, Fructus Lycii 20 to 30g

poilished round—grained rice, Semen Oryzae Sativae 60g

refined salt, Sal Communis a bit

scallion stalk, Bulbus Allii Fistulosi 2

fresh ginger, Rhizoma Zingiberis Recens 3 slices

PROCESS First, decoct the dodder seeds, raspberry and wolfberry fruit together in an earthenware pot to obtain medicinal extract and remove the dregs; have the sparrows rid of the feathers, the intestines and other internal organs, wash them clean and parch them in wine; cook the sparrows, rice and medicinal extract with addition of the right amount of water to make thin gruel. When it is about to be done, put in refined salt, scallion stalks and fresh ginger.

DIRECTIONS Take such gruel once in the morning and once in the evening, on an empty stomach.

EFFICACY Invigorating yang—qi, replenishing the essence and blood, tonifying the liver and kidney.

INDICATIONS Symptoms caused by deficiency of the kidney—qi such as impotence, seminal emission and premature emission, giddiness, dim eyesight, tinnitus and deafness, enuresis and, in women, leukorrhagia. For old people, it can improve health and prolong life if taken frequently over a long period of time.

PRECAUTIONS It is fit to be taken in winter, 3 to 5 days as a course of treatment. Those who have a fever or sexual hyperesthesia should not take it.

2) Life—Prolonging Soup of Pigeon Egg (Yishon Gedan Tang)

SOURCE Records of Chinese Materia Medica in Sichuan Province

INGREDIENTS

wolfberry fruit, Fructus Lycii 10g

longan aril, Arillus Longan 10g

prepared Siberian solomonseal rhizome, Rhizoma Polygonati Praeparata 10g

pigeon egg 4

crystal sugar 50g

PROCESS Have wolfberry fruit, longan aril and prepared Siberian solomonseal rhizome washed clean and cut into pieces; pound crystal sugar into bits and put them in a bowl. Put a pot on the fire, add about 750 ml of clean water into the pot; put in the three ingredients and boil them for about 15 minutes; beat the pigeon eggs and put them into the pot one by one; add crystal sugar bits and go on cooking until they are done.

DIRECTIONS Take it once a day, for seven days successively.

EFFICACY Replenishing the liver and kidney, tonifying qi and blood, moistening the lung and strengthening constitution.

INDICATIONS It has a relatively good curative effect upon symptoms such as cough due to dryness of the lung, deficiency of qi and blood, and failing of mentality, etc. It can also be used as health-care food for those who suffer from pain in the loins due to deficiency of the kidney, sallow complexion, emaciation, and senile debility.

（京）新登字 207 号

图书在版编目(CIP)数据

中华药膳＝MEDICATED DIET OF TRADITIONAL CHINESE MEDICINE/侯景伦主编．—北京：北京科学技术出版社，1994.12
ISBN 7-5304-1735-5

Ⅰ.中… Ⅱ.侯… Ⅲ.食物疗法—中国 Ⅳ.R247.1

中国版本图书馆 CIP 数据核字(94)第 15620 号

中 华 药 膳

主 编：侯景伦

副主编：赵 昕 李卫东

编 委：刘建新 耿春娥 李国华 李少华

北京科学技术出版社出版

（中国北京西直门南大街 16 号）

华燕印刷厂印刷

中国国际图书贸易总公司发行

（中国北京车公庄西路 35 号）

北京邮政信箱第 399 号 邮政编码 100044

1994 年 12 月第一版第一次印刷

英文版 16 开本

ISBN7-5304-1735-5/R・309

04850

14-E-2905P